ATHLETICS AND THE HEART

Athletics and the Heart

Dr. med. RICHARD ROST

Translated by

THOMAS J. DEKORNFELD, M.D.

YEAR BOOK MEDICAL PUBLISHERS, INC.
Chicago • London

1 2 3 4 5 6 7 8 9 C K 89 88 87 86

This book is an authorized translation from the German edition published and copyrighted 1984 by Perimed Fachbuch—Verlagsgesellschaft mbH, Erlangen, Germany. Title of the German edition: *Herz Und Sport*.

Library of Congress Cataloging-in-Publication Data

Rost, Richard.
    Athletics and the heart.
    Translation of: Herz und Sport.
    Includes bibliographies and index.
    1. Heart.   2. Sports—Physiological aspects.
3. Exercise—Physiological aspects.   4. Athletes—
Health and hygiene.   I. Title.   [DNLM: 1. Exertion.
2. Heart—physiology.   3. Sports.   4. Sports Medicine.
WG202 R839h]
RC1236.H43R6713   1986   612'.17   86-13179
ISBN 0-8151-7397-0

Sponsoring Editor: Linda A. Miller
Manager, Copyediting Services: Frances M. Perveiler
Copyeditor: Julie DuSablon
Production Project Manager: Max Perez
Proofroom Supervisor: Shirley E. Taylor

Contents

1

Introduction

The relationships between the heart and athletics are manifold, fascinating, and of increasing practical significance for all those who wish to become involved in this area. Even the etymological derivation of the word "heart" is significant. Not all cardiologists are aware of the fact that the subject of their professional and scientific interest received its name from an athletic term by our forefathers. According to Boyadijan, the word "heart" has the same indogermanic root as the word "hart" (male deer). This could perhaps be freely translated as "jumper," so named by early man because the heart was "jumping" in the chest after heavy exertion.

The amazing range of performance that the heart is capable of can best be seen in athletics. The work load of the heart is quadrupled and the cardiac output is raised from 5–6 L/minute to 20–25 L/minute. The trained heart can raise its performance eightfold to 40 L/minute. In the resting state cardiac action has to function only at the lower one-fourth of its potential.

Such a functional point of view has wide implications in areas other than the heart of the healthy, active person. Athletics are increasingly recognized as a therapeutic modality for cardiac patients and as a prophylactic measure in the prevention of cardiocirculatory problems. This is shown in the enormous increase of ambulatory coronary activity centers. In the past 5 years, their number has risen from 80 to 800 in the German Federal Republic alone. Furthermore, the significant advances in cardiac surgery have placed into an entirely new perspective the importance of athletics in the management of cardiac patients. Coronary bypass surgery, valvular replacement, and other surgical interventions improve the performance potential of the failing heart, but can come to full fruition only when physiotherapy and rehabilitation improve the performance of the entire body.

The increasing importance of athletics in the prophylaxis of cardiovascular disease and in the treatment of the cardiac patient has been sufficiently recognized so that interest in this area is no longer limited to a small group of specialists as it was in the 1960s. For decades, the sports-cardiologists were interested primarily, and with few exceptions, in the peculiarities and evaluation of the athlete's heart. There were only a few cardiologists who recognized the importance of athletics for the sick heart. These discussions, which extend almost over a century, have resulted in a number of findings that today form the basis for athletic activities in the cardiac patient.

Clinicians have always regarded the large and efficient heart of the athlete with suspicion, and there are cardiologists who even today consciously or instinctively consider the athlete's heart as a form of cardiomyopathy. Such a view is understandable when one looks at the characteristics of these hearts, e.g., the increase in size, the resting rate at or below 30 beats per minute, the appearance of unusual electrocardiograph (ECG) findings, such as functional third degree atrioventricular (AV) block, and reentry disturbances, which can simulate the findings seen in infarction. In spite of such findings, which raise a question about the range of physiologic adaptation of the heart, it must be emphasized that the decade-long discussions concerning the athlete's heart have proved only one thing: we are dealing with healthy and particularly effective hearts. The above-mentioned peculiarities of the athlete's heart and the importance of athletics for the cardiac patient make it necessary that the relationship between the heart and athletics become a major concern for the cardiologist. This need is not considered adequately in the standard textbooks on classical cardiology. The athlete's heart is either not mentioned at all or is largely discussed in a negative fashion. This is particularly true in the Anglo-American literature. In the more than 2,000-page textbook on cardiovascular medicine by Braunwald (1980), the words "athletics" or "athlete's heart" do not appear in the index. The ultimate in denial is reached by Friedberg (1972) who claims that the cardiac enlargement in the athlete may, among other interpretations, be due to overload on a heart previously damaged by syphilis.

Such gross misrepresentations cannot be found in the more recent German literature. This can certainly be attributed to Reindell (1960), who was an outstanding champion for the athlete's heart and who devoted the scholarly activities of a lifetime to the recognition that the athlete's heart was a positive adaptation phenomenon. Thanks to him and others, functionally oriented considerations of load and efficiency have been introduced

into modern cardiology that prior to this time were limited to "resting phase" considerations. In consequence, stress ECG, ergometry, and pulmonary artery pressure measurements under stress can be considered as standard procedures.

In spite of this progress, even today the scientific and practical significance of the relationship of athletics and the heart gets all but short shrift in German textbooks on cardiology. It must be remembered, in this context, that the coronary activity clubs developed largely outside the mainstream of clinical cardiology. To date, clinical cardiology has not paid enough attention to the impact of physical stress on the healthy and sick heart. For the clinical cardiologist, the cardiac patient is still a person lying in bed whose functional ability can be precisely analysed in a resting state, and whose differential response to different stress (running, swimming, weight training) need not be considered outside the hospital.

This lack of involvement of the clinical cardiologist with the effects of physical activity on cardiac function illustrates one of the general problems of sports medicine. In spite of the considerable importance granted today by society to both competitive sports and to mass participation in athletics, it has been impossible so far to establish an independent department of sports medicine at any university medical school. The physician is frequently asked questions by a patient who wishes to engage in physical activity because of his heart; questions that the physician can only answer unsatisfactorily.

The patient who engages in athletics for the benefit of his heart usually does so to prevent cardiocirculatory problems. The motivation for this activity is provided by mortality statistics that show cardiovascular disease causing more than 50% of all deaths, and by advertising slogans such as, "Run away from your heart attack!" Unfortunately, patients are also aware of the opposing opinions in this area, which are manifested by such contrary advice as, "Engage in sport *and* stay healthy" and "Engage in sport *or* stay healthy."

The motivation to write this monograph was provided by numerous colleagues who, during various postgraduate courses, expressed a wish to have a single volume in which they could review the relationships between athletics and the heart. Such a volume is currently not available in the literature. Since the last, and now classic, presentations of the Freiburg Group (Reindell, 1960) numerous new aspects of the athlete's heart and the general value of athletics to health have emerged. Even though the presentation of Reindell was considered to close the book on any further discussion of the athlete's heart, new noninvasive techniques, e.g., echocardiography, have brought new perspectives to bear on this issue. The newest developments in the area of athletics and cardiac patients were unforeseen 20 years ago.

For this reason it seems appropriate, once again, to determine the status of sports cardiology. To determine this status, it is necessary not only to review the scientific developments in this field, but also to realize the need to examine the relationships between athletics and the heart from a practical, medical point of view. An attempt will be made to answer the questions asked by patients from the practicing physician and which the latter usually passes on to the specialist in sports medicine. These answers will be approached from a scientific point of view.

The following subject areas will be discussed in detail:

1. The *way the heart functions* under the different forms of physiologic stress. The wide variety of athletic activities makes it understandable that the responses of the cardiocirculatory system will differ considerably from each other. The physician who is familiar with these relationships can respond to the different

signs and symptoms specifically on the basis of etiology.

2. The *adaptation responses* of the heart under physiologic stress. The athlete's heart will be described from the perspective of historical development and on the basis of its anatomic and clinical characteristics.

3. The *possible cardiac incidents* related to athletic activity. The most dramatic and affecting of these incidents is the sudden cardiac arrest. It is for this reason that particular medical attention must be directed toward the question of whether physiologic load can really lead to cardiac damage. The lay person usually accepts the health benefits of athletics as a matter of course but it is the duty of sports physician to determine the limits beyond which activity no longer contributes to health.

4. The value of athletics for the *cardiac patient* as a central issue in sports cardiology.

5. The necessary interaction of the therapeutic modalities, particularly the physical activity of the cardiac patient and the *pharmacologic management* of the same individual. While the relationship between these two therapeutic modalities has not been properly elucidated, it is desirable to highlight its particular significance.

It should be emphasized that athletics and medicine must work as partners in the care of cardiac patients. For that reason this volume is dedicated to the physician who is deeply concerned not only for the heart of the athletes but also for the heart of his other patients who engage in physical activity. This volume should be of particular benefit to athletic coaches and trainers who spend their life in this activity and whose duty it is to fit the trainees' performance into the framework established by the medical considerations.

2

Heart Action Under Physical Exercise

The human body is designed for muscular activity which can raise basal metabolism by a factor of 15 to 20.

P. Astrand, 1974

The range of circulatory performance becomes manifest only under physical exercise. The different types of exercise result in correspondingly different cardiocirculatory responses. The diversity of these reactions is generally only poorly known.

In order to illustrate this diversity and these contradictions, some extreme variations will be presented as follows: It is generally assumed that exercise raises the blood pressure and the cardiac output. In the untrained person this rise can be four- to fivefold; in the trained person the rise can be as much as eightfold when compared to the resting volume. These changes can take place, but are certainly not inevitable. Under maximal effort of a certain type, e.g., under maximal power load, the cardiac output can drop to half of the resting value. Mean blood pressure can remain unchanged, e.g., running on a level surface. It can also drop under certain conditions of maximal effort, or it can rise by several thousand mm Hg, for instance, as in diving.

To be able to classify the various responses and to try to derive some uni-formly applicable general laws concerning the various responses to physical effort, the two basic forms of muscular activity, isotonic and isometric contractions, will be taken as the starting point in the subsequent discussion. The shortening of the muscle fibers generally determines the dynamic work of the muscle, while the development of tension of the fibers determines the static holding work of the muscle. The two components of cardiac work, pressure and volume, will be discussed in the context of the above two forms of muscular activity. The data presented were partly generated by the author and partly derived from the literature. In as much as they are considered incomplete the reader is referred to an earlier, more complete presentation (Rost, 1979).

THE WORK OF THE HEART UNDER A DYNAMIC LOAD

The dynamic load is characterized by a rhythmic contraction and relaxation of muscle. In the athletic world it can be found in running, cross-country skiing, bicycle riding, swimming, and rowing. This sequence was selected on purpose. In the first types of exercise, the muscle contraction must closely approximate the physiologic nature of isotonia. In the subsequent types of exercise, an increasing force component becomes evident. Thus, in contrast to running, bicycle riding has a moderate, and rowing a pronounced, force component.

The dynamic contraction of the muscle may also manifest a certain, variable degree of tension development. This isometric muscle activity leads to a compression of extensive vascular fields, which clearly influences and affects the circulatory response, as discussed below. Let us start with a dynamic load, with minimal force development, as seen in running on level ground.

The *circulatory goal* is to transport more blood, i.e., to increase cardiac output. The extent of this rise can be determined accurately in a given individual, since it depends on the intensity of the performance, although it can be modified by such additional factors as body build, sex, age, and pathologic conditions.

The Cardiac Output

To be able to determine the increased work, the heart has to perform for a given effort, it must be assumed as a basic premise, that identical efforts require identical energy outputs. The efficiency of muscle is neither age- nor sex-dependent and cannot be improved by training. The unit of measurement for bodily performance is the watt. Every increase of one watt requires an increase in oxygen transport of 12 ml/minute. The energy requirement thus increases linearly with the intensity of load (Fig 2–1).

On the other hand, the pumping action of the heart increases linearly with the energy utilization. The relationship between the increase in oxygen uptake and cardiac output can be expressed as the so-called "exercise factor." It corresponds to the required increase in cardiac output for every 100 ml increase in

oxygen uptake and usually lies about 0.61. The precise relationship is expressed in the equation described by Holmgren (1956):

$$\text{Cardiac output (L/min)} = 7.03 + 0.0058 \times VO_2 \text{ (ml/min)}$$

This means that for a performance of 100 watt, 1.21 L/minute additional oxygen is required. To deliver this amount, the heart must increase its output by 7.2 L. Starting with a resting output of 6 L this means that the minute volume must rise to approximately 13 L for a 100-watt performance. A 200-watt performance requires a cardiac output of 20 L. We can also estimate the output required on the basis of the speed of running. In level running the power cannot be expressed in watts, since according to the following formula, at least in theory:

$$\text{Power} = \text{Force} \times \text{distance/time}$$

Therefore, since no height has to be overcome, the power must equal zero. The required minute volume, however, can be derived from the required energy utilization. Oxygen uptake can be calculated for a given speed of running, by an equation according to Pugh (1970):

$$VO_2 \text{ (ml/min} \times \text{kg)} = 4.25 + 2.98 \times \text{speed (km/hr)}$$

The *regulation of cardiac output* on the basis of demand is one of the central topics of circulatory physiology under conditions of physical exercise. There are as many theories as there are investigators. In principle, all these theories can be divided into two groups. According to one theory, the heart as an active muscle regulates itself. If an increase in flow is required, the heart increases its output and this secondarily increases venous return. The contrary view claims that the heart is the "servant" of the circulation, and that the cardiac output is largely determined by the amount of venous return. Accordingly, cardiac performance is de-

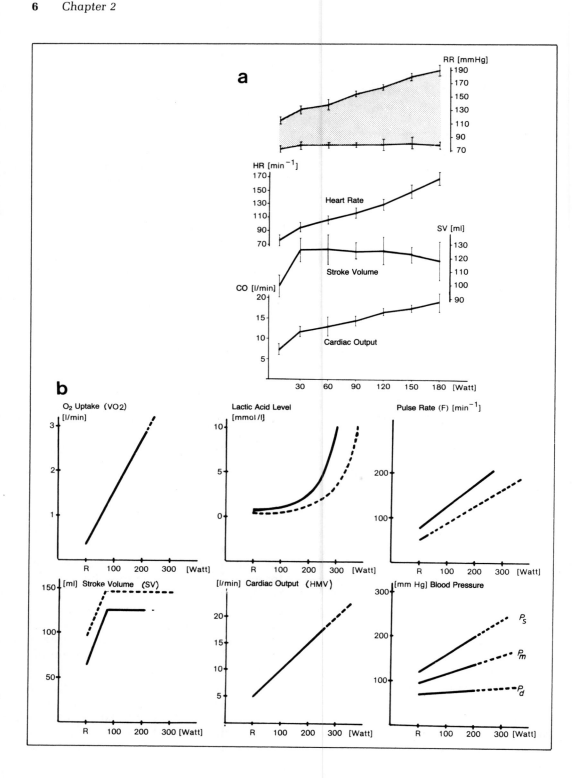

termined by the conditions in the periphery.

Such a division appears to be artificial. Factors that affect the cardiac output automatically alter venous return and vice versa. The control system of the circulation is a complex equilibrium, in which the metabolic requirements of all the organs participate, and that is affected by numerous humoral, nervous, and mechanical control mechanisms. The change in one factor leads retroactively to changes in other systems.

Possible control mechanisms were identified in cortical reflexes, humeral impulses, chemoreceptors, and pressoreceptors. Cortical impulses do play a role in the adaptation to load conditions as shown in the *prestart reaction*. Runners show an appreciable increase in pulse rate and blood pressure even before the start, which provide an increased blood supply to the muscles. On the other hand, such a mechanism cannot provide a precise control under load conditions.

The theory of adaptation on the basis of *reflex self regulation* by Koch (1931)

was previously widely accepted. According to this theory, the start of any physical exercise or increase of intensity leads to a dilatation of the vessels in the periphery and to a central fall in pressure. This should lead to a reflex increase in cardiac performance via the baroreceptors in the great vessels, e.g., in the carotid sinus. Direct arterial blood pressure measurement failed to show such a central drop in blood pressure at the onset of exercise. Even the *Bainbridge reflex* was considered to be responsible for the increase in cardiac performance through a reflex response to increased atrial filling.

Adaptation of the circulation to conditions of load can be readily explained on the basis of a peripheral muscular regulatory mechanism. Alam and Smirk (1937) have shown that regulation of the blood pressure during exercise could be effected by peripheral muscles via the chemoreceptors and mechanoreceptors. Stegeman (1974) developed a theory that based the regulation of circulation primarily on muscular chemoreceptors. If the metabolic conditions in the muscle

---

FIG 2–1.

Circulatory responses under dynamic load. **a,** hemodynamic measurements obtained in five volunteers in the supine position with increasing loads using the dye-dilution technique. While cardiac output and pulse rate increase in a linear fashion with increasing loads, the stroke volume increases initially but then remains level in spite of increasing loads. Blood pressure was measured by the indirect method in this study. The increase in diastolic pressure found by direct arterial pressure measurements (see Fig 2–3,B), cannot be seen in this study. **b,** the findings in the area of energy production and circulatory adaptation are compared between trained and nontrained volunteers in a schematic fashion. The *solid line* represents the values obtained in the nontrained. The *broken line* represents the comparable values in the trained persons. With increasing loads, there is a linear increase in energy production over oxygen consumption *(upper left)*. The trained athlete consumes the same amount of oxygen for the same amount of load, although he can reach load levels that are beyond the capacity of the nontrained person. The sec-

ond important factor in energy utilization is the production of lactic acid. Initially no lactic acid is produced, but there is a sharp increase in lactic acid values at the two-third mark of maximal effort (aerobic-anaerobic threshold). This curve is shifted to the right in the trained athlete *(upper center)*. The rise in oxygen consumption is based on a corresponding increase in cardiac output *(lower center)*. Here again there is an identical cardiac output per load level for both the trained and nontrained person. The two components of cardiac output, i.e., the pulse rate and the stroke volume, are shown on the *upper right* and *lower left side,* respectively. Since the trained athlete has a larger stroke volume, he can get by with a lower pulse rate for an identical load intensity. The maximal pulse rate, which is about the same as in the nontrained person, is reached only at levels of load intensity that are beyond the capacity of the nontrained person. The blood pressure values are the same in the trained and nontrained at similar intensities of load.

deteriorate—the specific metabolic stimulus has not yet been identified—this results in an increased sympathetic drive of the heart and a corresponding increase in cardiocirculatory performance.

Even though the regulatory mechanism has not been fully elucidated, there is an adaptation of the heart to increased load that is based on an increased sympathetic tone, i.e., on an extracardiac mechanism.

The intracardiac reserves of the heart, the so-called *Starling mechanism*, are significant only in adaptations to momentary swings in demand. The fact that the Starling mechanism does not play a significant role in the adaptation of the heart to performance requirements can be seen from the observation that during exercise the end-diastolic ventricular filling changes just as little as the filling pressure.

The significance of the Starling mechanism on the athlete's heart will be discussed further in the section on "Function of the Athlete's Heart."

Of the two components of the cardiac output, heart rate and stroke volume, heart rate is the significant factor in the adaptation to performance. The anatomic configuration of the ventricle is the limiting factor in the ability to increase stroke volume. When the muscular pumping action begins to increase, there will be an increase in venous return and some increase in stroke volume. Further increase in activity, however, does not lead to further increase in stroke volume. An increase in inotropy under sympathetic stimulation leads to an increase in stroke volume. It can be shown by echocardiography that identical diastolic filling still allows an increase in systolic output (see Fig 3–15). While pulse rate, output, and oxygen consumption increase linearly with the intensity of load, the *stroke volume* behaves fundamentally differently, as shown in Figure 2–1.

The degree of increase in stroke volume depends on body position. Most of the existing studies were performed with the subject in the supine position. Under these circumstances the dye-dilution technique shows a 25% increase in stroke volume, while studies using the Fick principle show an increase of only 10%. Studies with the subject in the sitting position show an increase in stroke volume of 30% to 50%. In studies performed on a treadmill, i.e., with the subject in the standing position, Hanson (1965) and Wang (1960) have found an increase in the stroke volume of 100%. These differences can be attributed to the decreased resting stroke volume normally found in the standing position. This orthostatic effect is compensated for by the muscle pump.

According to some data in the literature, particularly the findings of Bevegard (1963), the muscle pump is insufficient to fully compensate for the *orthostatic effect*. According to these findings, the cardiac output in the sitting position is 1 to 2 L less than in the supine position, given the same load. Our own comparative studies could not reproduce these findings. In our studies, cardiac output was identical in the sitting and supine position during bicycle ergometry.

Interestingly, the highest stroke volume is attained not during the exercise but immediately afterwards. This is due to the fact that immediately following the cessation of exercise, the pulse rate drops very rapidly, while the venous return remains very high. In this situation, the already mentioned *Starling mechanism* plays an important stop-gap role. The increase in stroke volume can last for about 3 minutes beyond the maximal stress, and is dependent upon the intensity of the load.

These relationships are primarily of historic interest, since in the 1950s they served to establish the *short-term-interval-training* even for endurance athletes. The assumption was that the increase in stroke volume was the determinant stimulus for the enlargement of the heart, and therefore, the shortest possible load-times and correspondingly frequent intervals during the same training period, allowed a large number of the so-called "reward pauses." This led to the practice that even long distance runners had to undergo short distance training and were running 20 consecutive 200 meter dashes. The fact that this assumption was ultimately found to be wrong is based on the finding that endurance training cannot be viewed from a hemodynamic perspective. It also ignored the effects of training on the metabolic mechanisms that have such decisive importance in the athlete conditioned for sustained effort.

In contrast to stroke volume, the *heart rate* has a decisive effect on the fine adaptation of cardiac performance to stress. While the stroke volume in the untrained person can rise from 80 ml in supine position and 60 ml in the standing position to only 100–120 ml under maximal exercise, the heart can triple its rate, from 70 beats per minute to 200 beats per minute under similar conditions. Thus, the *maximal cardiac output* can be raised from 20 L to 25 L in the untrained person. The *maximal heart rate* is determined biologically and is age dependent, but not sex or training dependent. As rule of thumb, the average value for maximal heart rate can be taken as 220/minute minus age. Thus in a 10-year-old child it will be 210 beats per minute and in a 40-year-old person, 180 beats per minute. The two standard deviations of this value is ± 20. In youngsters, therefore, a maximal value of 230 can be reached. Higher maximal rates, e.g., 250 and even 300, which are occasionally reported by athletes, are usually due to counting errors. We were never able to demonstrate such values by Holter monitoring. A threefold increase in pulse rate is necessarily conditional on a shortening of the contractile process. This is evident

from an *increase in contractility*. Studies by Roskamm (1972) (see Fig 3–16) have shown that in the untrained person the maximal rate of pressure increase can be quintupled as a parameter of contractility.

In setting the cardiac output volume for a given exercise, the available circulating *blood volume* must increase its rate of flow. The blood volume reserves that, according to Wollheim (1931), can be mobilized in response to stress in animals from the splenic and hepatic reservoir, do not exist in man. In fact, the available blood volume decreases by about 5% under load conditions. This is the result of the appearance of hemoconcentration. *Hemoglobin values* can increase 1–2 gm% under stress, as consequence of the decrease in plasma volume. Several mechanisms participate in this occurrence, e.g., an increase in filtration pressure, as a consequence of increased blood pressure, and an increase in capillary permeability (see Ekelund, 1967; Kirsch, 1968).

In order to have a clearer understanding of the time factor in this acceleration of the blood volume, reference must be made to the *steady state* concept. In every discussion concerning the achievement of an optimal exercise in the context of ergometry, it is emphasized that the duration of the exercise must be at least 6 minutes per watt step increase. Only such a time span can reasonably assure the establishment of an appropriate equilibrium. It is in fact mandatory that such a time sequence be maintained in order to accelerate the sluggish blood mass from a circulating volume of 5 to 6 L/minute to the maximal or submaximal cardiac output. Our own studies have shown that the time-volume rate required for a 200-watt load could not be achieved in 3 minutes but could be achieved in 6 minutes. It remained constant thereafter, in spite of increased load-time. This time span of 5 to 6 minutes to establish the steady state cannot be extrapolated to minor increases in load. If a performance of 25 watt is required, this means an increase in cardiac output from a 6 L/minute to 8 L/minute. This increase can be achieved in 1 to 2 minutes so that after this time span the required cardiac output is obtained.

If the time of exercise is extended once the steady state value has been achieved, the cardiac output remains generally constant. In hemodynamic studies, Ekelund (1967) found that with exercise times of up to 30 minutes there was a continuous increase in heart rate, but that the cardiac output remained stable once the steady state had been reached. This means that increasing exercise times are accompanied by a decrease in stroke volume. This relationship can be explained well by the regulatory mechanism postulated by Stegemann (1974). Increasing exercise time leads to a deterioration of the metabolic status in the muscle, which leads to an increased sympathetic drive, and thus to an increase in heart rate. Since the venous return does not increase appreciably, the stroke volume must decrease.

Finally it must be mentioned that the established cardiac output does depend on *age* and *sex*. With the exception of the known facts relating to the elderly, the data in the literature are poor. Astrand (1964) claimed that in the *female* the cardiac output was higher for a given load. He assumes that this is due to lower hemoglobin concentration. This hypothesis is not supported by other data, and Musshoff (1959) found no difference in exercise cardiac output between males and females. A lower hemoglobin value means a decrease in the maximal *arteriovenous oxygen gradient*. It does not, however, necessarily mean a decreased oxygen utilization at submaximal effort. Naturally females must produce a higher heart rate than males, given the same level of exercise, because of their generally smaller heart size and smaller stroke volume.

As far as the effect of age on exercise cardiac output is concerned, there are for obvious reasons, very few data in *children* based on invasive measurement techniques. According to the findings of Erikson (1971) the cardiac output in children is less than in adults for comparable loads. This finding needs to be substantiated by further studies. A decrease in cardiac output in the *elderly*, however, has been clearly demonstrated in conditions of equal loads. In this respect, the findings of Granath (1964) are particularly pertinent. The cardiac output and oxygen uptake is about 1 to 2 L/min less for similar loads than in the younger person. The peripheral oxygen utilization, however, is correspondingly increased. Since in the elderly, sclerotic changes lead to an increase in mean arterial pressure under similar loads, there is a shift in cardiac work during exercise from volume-work to pressure-work, even though the total cardiac work remains approximately the same. According to the studies of Gollwitzer-Meier (1937) this is an undesirable development since pressure work is much more detrimental for myocardial oxygen requirements than volume work.

Arterial Pressure

The final comments of the previous section introduce one of the significant components of cardiac work under stress, namely arterial pressure, that will be discussed in detail below. The behavior of blood pressure is quite variable and can undergo rapid changes, as compared to the much more sluggish changes in cardiac output. These conditions could be elucidated only when direct arterial pressure measurements became available and when telemetry became a practical tool. In this relationship, the studies of Bachmann (1969, 1970) are particularly pertinent.

The comments concerning the usefulness of direct arterial pressure measurements, lead naturally into some remarks concerning the *indirect blood pressure measurement, or Riva-Rocci, method.* This latter method allows only a very limited understanding of the behavior of pressure under stress. On one hand the method is very slow, and stretches over a number of heart beats, so that rapid changes cannot be appreciated. On the other hand, this method is very unreliable in determining the diastolic pressure and thus makes the determination of mean pressure equally unreliable. Ergometric studies have shown that when diastolic pressure was measured by the indirect method, it frequently showed a decrease under increasing stress. In extreme cases, it is sometimes possible to observe the so-called *null phenomenon* when, usually after stress, the Korotkoff sounds were audible even though the cuff pressure had fallen to zero. Comparative, direct, and indirect measurements do not support such observations (Fig 2–

2). According to direct measurements on the bicycle ergometer, increasing stress results in increasing diastolic pressure, although to a lesser degree than the systolic pressure.

The decrease in diastolic pressure, found frequently with indirect pressure measurements during bicycle ergometry, does not correspond to the true conditions existing in the vascular tree. The basis for the original observation was a problem of technique. To date, there is no generally accepted theory concerning the origin of the Korotkoff sounds or why these sounds disappear in the neighborhood of the diastolic pressure, or indeed what the precise criteria are for the measurement of diastolic pressure. The recommendations whether to use the decline in the sounds (phase IV) or the disappearance of the sounds (phase V) vary from expert to expert. Nevertheless, it can be stated that the origin of the Korotkoff sounds is related to intravascular flow and to the pressure of the cuff. Under stress, the intravascular flow is in-

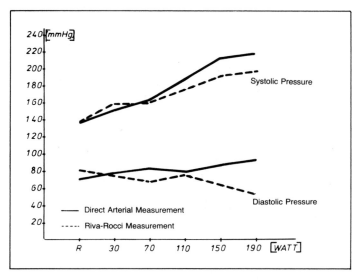

FIG 2–2.

Comparison of arterial pressure obtained by direct and indirect measurement during ergometry. The systolic pressure is very similar by both techniques. On the other hand, the diastolic pressure shows an apparent decline with increasing loads when measured by the Riva-Rocci method. This finding cannot be substantiated by direct arterial measurement.

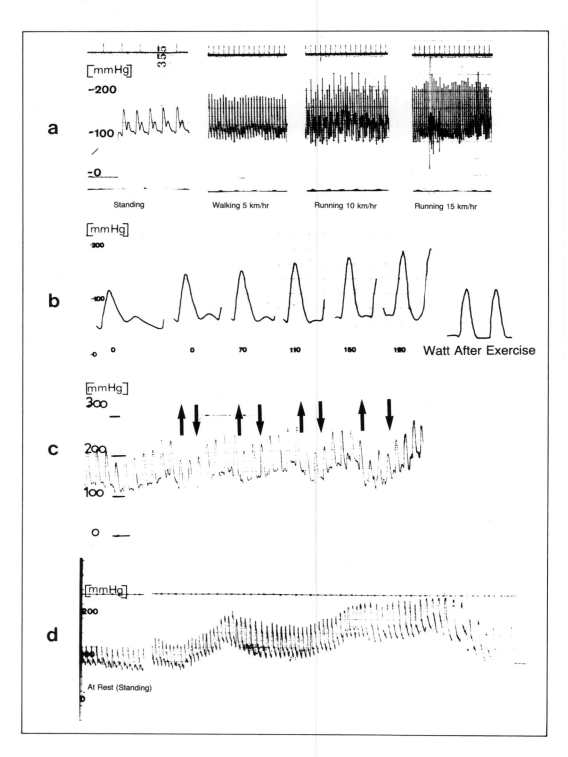

creased to the point where the pressure of the stethoscope suffices to produce sounds, even though the cuff pressure has fallen to zero.

Because of the lack of reliability of the indirect method, *direct pressure measurements under stress* have revealed new and surprising results. Since an increase in pressure under physical exercise was first described by Zadek (1881), it has been considered self-evident that physical activity results in an increase in blood pressure. This does not seem to be obvious when looked at teleologically. If the goal of the circulation during exercise is to increase the cardiac output, the flow, and the amount of oxygen carried, this could be accomplished, according to Ohm's law, without increase in pressure and solely through a corresponding decrease in peripheral resistance. It does not seem apparent why the heart should have to increase its pressure-work substantially just to increase the amount of blood pumped.

From the point of view of circulatory economy, the most sensible solution would be if an increase in cardiac output were compensated for by a corresponding dilatation of the blood vessels. It will come as a surprise to those who are not particularly knowledgeable in circulatory dynamics during exercise that if the load

is primarily due to isotonic muscle contractions, the above-described circulatory model is closely approximated. Thus, in running, the mean arterial pressure does not rise significantly, as proved by arterial pressure curves. It is shown in Figure 2–3 that during *running* with increasing speed, the diastolic pressure remains unchanged, while the systolic pressure rises. Figure 2–3 also shows that there is a simultaneous distortion of the pressure wave form. The dicrotic wave keeps sliding lower and lower. Since during running the shaking of the indwelling catheter makes it almost impossible to get artifact-free tracings, the changes in the pressure wave form have been substantiated during pedaling exercises in the supine position. Figure 2–3 shows in tracings obtained by this method that the dicrotic wave practically disappears with increasing stress and the arterial pressure curve becomes steeper.

Holmgren (1956) was the first one to point out this relationship. The change in the shape of the arterial curve is due to the decrease in peripheral resistance under stress and to the altered reflective responses in the periphery, which are responsible for the dicrotic wave. The *dicrotic phenomenon* is due to a superimposition of a "standing wave" on the pressure curve, which changes its maxi-

FIG 2–3.
Arterial pressure tracings under different types of dynamic exercises. **a,** arterial pressure while standing, walking, and running at two different speeds. The time markers show that the paper speed was reduced during running in order to capture more pressure waves. There is a speed-dependent increase in systolic pressure while the diastolic pressure remains unchanged. The dicrotic notches appear as a dark heavy line. This represents an increasing flattening of the dicrotic wave, seen better in **b. b,** bicycle ergometric exercises in the supine position. To illustrate the increasing steepness of the pressure wave better, a single wave is shown, obtained at a fast paper speed. A distinct rise in systolic pressure and a moderate rise in diastolic pressure can be seen. The di-

crotic pressure wave gradually flattens and is totally flat immediately after the end of the exercise. **c,** arterial pressures during push-ups. At the beginning of the push *(arrow pointing down),* there is a definite increase in pressure. When the arms are extended *(arrow pointing up),* the muscles relax. The decreased effort leads to an immediate drop in pressure. **d,** arterial pressure during diving. The measurements were made in a volunteer at a depth of 1 m. In order to avoid any Valsalva effect, the volunteer was equipped with a respirator. There is an increase in arterial pressure that corresponds to the external hydrostatic pressure (about 75 mm Hg). There is a simultaneous decrease in heart rate that corresponds to the increase in pulse pressure.

mum and minimum under stress. Even under resting conditions the systolic pressure wave is steeper in the brachial artery than in the aorta, and the systolic pressure is higher. In running, the central pressure does not rise appreciably and neither does the peripherally measured mean arterial pressure, which is a critical measure of the work of the heart. At the same time the systolic pressure appears to be significantly raised by a distortion of the wave form, described above.

These relationships make it very clear that the indirect peripheral blood pressure measurements give only very incomplete information concerning the true state of blood pressure and that assessment of the mean arterial pressure, purely on the basis of systolic pressure, leads to totally erroneous conclusions. On this basis the benefits of running and of similar exercises for the coronary artery patient and for the hypertensive patient become apparent. On the one hand, running, as a typical endurance exercise, has very beneficial training effects, on the other hand, running does not have to be "paid" for by a sustained increase in pressure that would increase the myocardial oxygen requirements unnecessarily.

An inspection of Figure 2–3 reveals, however, that when pedaling in the supine position, both the systolic and diastolic pressure rise, which necessarily leads to a rise in mean pressure. *Pedaling in the supine position* differs from running, in that it requires a considerably increased muscular force. In this exercise relatively large vascular fields are compressed by muscle activity, which prevents a dilatation of the vessels. Therefore, peripheral resistance cannot fall to the degree required by the increase in blood flow to the muscles. It follows from this observation that an athletic exercise will lead to increasing pressure parallel to increasing muscular force. *Pedaling in the sitting position* leads to a slight increase in pressure, since the amount of muscular strength in this position is con-

siderably less than in the supine position. The bicycle rider can use his entire body in the sitting position and thus save on muscular effort. For this reason bicycle riding can also be recommended to the already-mentioned groups of cardiocirculatory patients.

A rhythmical performance of *push-ups* constitutes a dynamic stress, requiring very high muscular force. It can be seen in Figure 2–3 that the arm flexion part of the push-up requires very great isometric work and that the pressure, in this phase of the exercise, can rise to 250 mm Hg. During the extension phase of the push-up, this increase disappears promptly. Almost identical curves were found during *rowing* exercises by Fleischer (1976), since in this exercise there is also a rhythmical alteration in isometric work. These forms of exercise are unsuitable for the patients who had an infarct or who are hypertensive.

High arterial pressure, as a consequence of concentrated effort is due to a superimposition of external forces upon the cardiocirculatory system. Similar forces can become operative under other circumstances, such as the pressure of a Valsalva maneuver, the presence of sudden acceleration or deceleration forces, or hydrostatic pressure.

The last example can be seen during *swimming* or *diving*. Because of the great interest in swimming as a tool in cardiac rehabilitation, the hemodynamic consideration of immersion and, particularly their pressure relationships, will be discussed in detail. Figure 2–3 shows the pressure curves recorded in a volunteer during immersion in water. It shows that the arterial pressure rises in parallel with the depth of immersion. In this way astonishing absolute pressure levels can be reached, as shown in an experimental model. When, during a world record attempt at free diving, the depth of 100 meters was reached, the entire body of the diver was exposed to an external pressure of 10 ATA (atmospheric pressure, absolute). The zero line in the right atrium is therefore raised to 7600 mm Hg and the blood pressure of the diver, measured against external conditions, reaches absolutely maximal levels. Even at a diving depth of 1 meter, absolute pressure rises by 0.1 ATA, i.e., 75 mm Hg. This would mean that the starting pressure of 130/80 is raised to 205/155.

These stunningly high pressures are imposed passively by the external hydrostatic pressure and do not have to be generated internally by the heart. Yet, immersion in water leads to other physiologic manifestations, which are important in the assessment of swimming in the context of athletic activities for the cardiac patient. As seen in Figure 2–3, diving leads to a definite bradycardia with a corresponding rise in the amplitude of pressure.

This decrease in heart rate is known as "*diver bradycardia.*" It constitutes an interesting phenomenon. According to a general survey of literature by Stegemann (1969), this bradycardia is an economy measure that permits a longer stay under water. In aquatic mammals it is very strongly developed; in man it is present only in a rudimentary form. Besides the development of a bradycardia, there are also other circulatory adjustments, namely a centralization of perfusion to the vital organs, the heart, and the brain. The diver bradycardia is triggered by the vagus and can be blocked by atropine. The mechanism that triggers the reflex is not clear. The etiology of an increased venous return due to the weightlessness in water, oxygen deficit, the Valsalva mechanism, and a trigeminal nerve receptor mechanism have all been proposed and may well operate in combination. The diver bradycardia can reach extreme levels. Figure 2–4 shows an example where the heart rate of a diver at 5 meters, measured telemetrically, dropped from his normal 70 beats per minute to 34 beats per minute. According to Stegemann, the diving reflex has such an effect on circulation that it overrides all other effects. Even the stress tachycardia is correspondingly reduced.

Data concerning the *cardiac rate* and *stroke volume* during swimming are rarely found in the literature because of

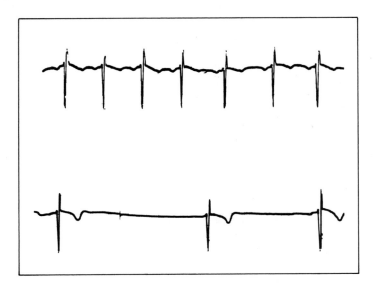

FIG 2–4.
ECG in a swimmer on the surface *(upper tracing)* and at 5 m depth *(lower tracing)*. The tracings were obtained by telemetry. The underwater heart rate of 34 beats per minute as compared to a surface rate of 70 beats per minute is an impressive demonstration of the diver bradycardia. (Recorded by Völker, 1983.)

the technical difficulties in obtaining them. Among the few available data, those of Holmer (1974) must be considered to be the most accurate ones, since they were obtained in five volunteers by the dye-dilution tehnique. A comparison of running and swimming shows that for equal oxygen uptake, the cardiac output, the stroke volume, and the heart rate are the same, but that the mean arterial pressure is 20 mm Hg higher in swimming.

According to these data, the characteristics of stress in water, such as hydrostatic pressure, work with the body in the horizontal position, the limitations placed on respiratory movements, and the higher heat conduction potential of water, have only a slight effect on the volume-work of the heart. In the area of maximal effort there is a decrease in comparison to running that lies in the neighborhood of 10%–20% for maximal oxygen utilization, maximal arteriovenous oxygen difference, and maximal heart rate. The maximal stroke volume remains unchanged, just as it does in submaximal ergometric stress measurements. These data also suggest that in swimming, as compared to running, the maximal cardiopulmonary capacity is decreased, since only a smaller percentage of the total muscle mass can be brought into play. It seems likely that the "weightlessness" plays a role, since those muscles that are used ordinarily to maintain the erect posture in a gravity field are not used in this situation. On the basis of these hemodynamic findings it can be expected that swimming will have a smaller effect on cardiopulmonary training than running.

The circulatory responses to dynamic stress are also affected by *individual factors,* in addition to the already mentioned factors of stress intensity, the proportion of isometric to isotonic muscle activity, and external pressure. Such individual factors include the highly individual psychologic response to a competitive situation, age, and the presence of pathologic changes. Figure 2–5 shows that, given the same stress, arterial pressure rises higher in the elderly, probably because of sclerotic changes. Concerning the shift from volume-work to pressure-work in the elderly, as shown in the studies of Granath (1964), the reader is referred to the previous section on "Cardiac Output."

In patients with hypertensive circulatory disturbances, the blood pressure elevations are significantly higher under conditions of stress. The resting pressure is only conditionally related to the stress hypertension. The latter has received considerable attention recently (Franz, 1979). The measurement of exercise blood pressure is particularly important in the hypertensive patient engaging in any form of athletics.

THE WORK OF THE HEART UNDER A STATIC LOAD

Sustained holding effort is characterized by isometric muscular contraction, i.e., by a pure rise in tension. It leads to a fundamentally different circulatory response than dynamic stress, since the intermittent muscular relaxation between two contractions is absent. Because of the tetanic, sustained contraction of the muscles, a paradoxical situation develops, as far as energy transport is concerned. On the one hand the muscle requires more energy, i.e., more available oxygen, on the other hand the activity of the muscle itself compromises the small intramuscular vessels and thus affects the transport of the required oxygen. This paradox of static muscular activity has been known since 1877 and was first described by *Gaskell.* In maximal force generation, the circulatory status is further complicated by the presence of the pressure squeeze generated by the so-called Valsalva maneuver.

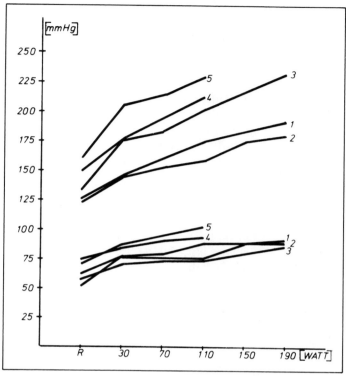

FIG 2–5.

Arterial pressures during ergometric exercises. The data were obtained by direct arterial measurements. Group 1 represents young, nontrained men; group 2 represents young, endurance-trained men; group 3 represents the findings in young, hypertensive men; group 4 represents older, nontrained men; and group 5 is values obtained from older, hypertensive men.

Submaximal Static Stress

In the following section the hemodynamic responses to submaximal load, i.e., without the presence of pressure squeezing, will be described. According to the findings of Lind and his associates, who have devoted particular study to this matter, the tension of the muscle must be below 15% of its maximal level to assure a sufficient perfusion of the muscle to meet the aerobic energy requirements. Above 70% of maximal tension, perfusion of the muscle may cease entirely. For this reason, static muscle work is determined almost entirely by anaerobic metabolism, mainly through the formation of lactic acid. A simple exercise can illustrate this point. Holding a chair at arms' length makes it quickly clear that such an anaerobic load can be sustained only for a short time, since the available anaerobic energy is limited. In addition, the developing lactic acid causes discomfort and, if there is excessive acid, enzymatic blockade ensues and all energy production ceases.

The circulatory response to such a static exercise is the exact opposite from the one described for a type of stress that is primarily due to isotonic muscle contraction, e.g., running. While the latter is characterized by a high volume-work and a low or absent increase in pressure, in isometric muscle work we find only a slight increase in the volume work of the heart, but a marked increase in pressure work. This model is readily understandable on a teleologic basis. An increase in *cardiac output* would make no sense since the working muscle is effectively excluded from the circulation. The purpose for the marked increase in pressure can be seen as an attempt by the circulation to counteract the transmural compression of the vessels by the muscle, and to provide the muscle with as much blood as these unfavorable conditions permit.

Our data, which agree with the above mentioned findings of Lind, show that during this type of holding work, cardiac output rises only to 10–12 L/minute. This is accomplished by an increase in heart rate to 120/minute, while the stroke volume remains the same. Since the peripheral resistance does not change either, the increase in cardiac output is sufficient to *raise the pressure* proportionately to the intensity of the holding-work. This can be seen clearly in arterial pressure tracings (Fig 2–6). In static stress, e.g., stretching a coil expander, the pressure can rise to 200/120 mm Hg. Examination of the pressure curves shows no distortion of the tracings, as it appears under dynamic stress. This is due to the fact that the change in the shape of the curve is due to changes in peripheral resistance that do not occur under static stress.

The circulatory conditions, as described, seem to be in contradiction to our original premise. Compression of the intramuscular vessels should lead to an increase in *peripheral resistance,* as had been described by Hettinger (1973). We must consider here, however, the opposing regulatory effects of the sympathetic nervous system. Through the activity of receptors, postulated to be present in muscle by Stegemann (1974), there is an increase in sympathetic tone. This leads to an increase in venous tone and thus to an increase in venous return to the heart. This, in turn, leads to an increase in cardiac output, the effect of which we can see as described in an increase in pres-

sure. The fact that the peripheral resistance does not rise, in spite of partial vascular compression, can be explained by a decrease in peripheral resistance in the nonworking muscles (Eklund, 1974). Under dynamic stress, the increase in pressure could be explained by a transmission of muscular compression effects to the larger vessels. In static holding work, which extends over a longer period of time, another component, a nervous reflex, also comes into play. Such reflexes in the autonomic system take several seconds to develop. This makes it impossible to explain the rise in pressure that parallels the exertion, as seen in Figure 2–3,C (push-ups) on this basis. In pure isometric work, however, that extends over a period of time, such reflexes are clearly operative. This is also demonstrated by the findings of Lind (1967) that show, that in static holding work, the rise in pressure depends on the percent participation of the individual muscles and not on the total muscle mass engaged in the exercise. A load of 50% of maximal effort on the great muscle mass of the leg results in the same rise of pressure as a 50% of maximal effort load on the very much smaller muscle mass of the arm. From a circulatory physiology point of view, it makes sense to distribute a static work load among the largest possible muscle mass to decrease the relative load on individual muscle fibers and to decrease the sympathetic stimulation of the heart.

The hemodynamic conditions, as described, explain why weight-load exercises are considered to be very unsuitable for the patient with organic cardiocirculatory disease. On the one hand, only those stimuli are effective in raising the performance of the cardiocirculatory system that result in an appropriate increase in cardiac output and that, according to Hollmann (1965), persist for at least 5 to 10 minutes, as it happens with dynamic stress. Static stress, therefore, is of no use

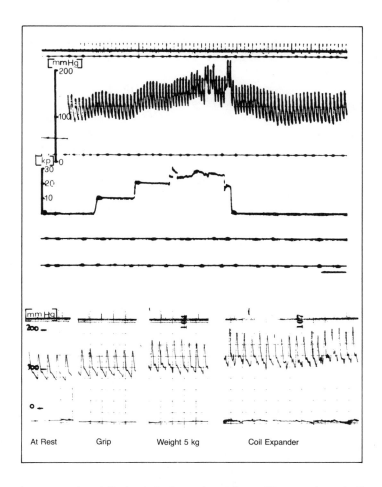

At Rest   Grip   Weight 5 kg   Coil Expander

FIG 2–6.

Arterial pressure changes under static load. In the upper part of the figure the effect of a hand grip-squeeze is shown by direct arterial measurement. The force generated is shown below the pressure tracing. The rise in pressure is parallel to the force generated. The highest tolerated load could be maintained by the subject just below the maximal energy output. The pressure curve accordingly is a typical example of the blood pressure tracings obtained un-der such conditions as shown in Figure 2–7. Contrary to the tracing shown in Figure 2–3, there is no change in the wave form, since there is no change in peripheral resistance. The *lower tracing* shows the response of the blood pressure to different forms of athletic stress. The expander-coil exercise raises the blood pressure from 130/80 mm Hg to 200/120 mm Hg.

in the training of the circulatory system and the sharp increase in pressure it engenders may be dangerous for the coronary or hypertensive patient.

On the other hand, we have to point out at this time that it would be a mistake to view the activities of the cardiocirculatory patient purely from the perspective of his current circulatory status. Even the circulatory patient needs muscles, which must be developed sensibly. In fact, a sensible muscular development training program for the cardiocirculatory patient can be based logically on the circulatory conditions described above. If the musculature is but poorly developed, even the slightest muscular demands of daily living will lead to a high tension state of the individual muscle fibers and thus to a significant sympathetic stimulus. For this reason, even the coronary patient should undergo some muscle conditioning. This should always be done, however, in the context of the desired maximal force and should, for didactic reasons, never exceed 50% of the theoretical maximum.

While weight-load exercises should be viewed with great caution in the patient with organic cardiocirculatory disease, the reverse is true for the hypotensive patient. For this patient weight-load exercises should be recommended that will raise the blood pressure and that will help to adapt the circulation to a more normal pressure regulation.

The Valsalva Maneuver

The circulatory response changes markedly under maximal weight-load stress because of the superimposition of an external pressure-squeeze. The *Valsalva maneuver* is a reflex phenomenon that is utilized in a variety of ways and means other than weight-loading, in such varied circumstances as defecation, child birth, trumpet blowing, recompressing the inner ear, etc. The purpose of this mechanism, consisting of an increase in intrathoracic pressure, achieved by exhaling against the closed glottis, is to establish the most stable base for the insertion and origin of the muscles of the thorax and spinal column. The *intrathoracic pressure* that can be generated by this maneuver is very high. Through telemetry we have seen central venous pressures as high as 178 mm Hg in weight lifters (Fig 2–8). In this kind of straining intrathoracic pressure can be assumed to rise by 100 to 200 mm Hg.

This increase in intrathoracic pressure leads to a dramatic interference with venous return that can be observed clearly in the distention of the neck veins. Our own studies have shown that in response the *cardiac output* is decreased by half of its original level. Since there is a simultaneous reflex increase in *heart rate*, the *stroke volume* can fall to a third of its normal value. This lowering of the stroke volume is shown echocardiographically in Figure 2–7. Such images can graphically illustrate the concept of the "empty beating" of the heart under weight-load stress as described in the older literature. In fact, a true "empty beating" heart never occurs. The blood content of the thorax and abdomen, which here function as a unit, is so great that during the 20–30 seconds that is the maximum period for which a Valsalva maneuver can be sustained, the heart can never really become "empty."

The imposition of pressure on the circulation results in some interesting changes in the *arterial pressure* curve, described for the first time by Hamilton (1936) and illustrated in Figure 2–7. First there is a pressure peak, which is the result of the superimposition of the pressure-squeeze on the arterial pressure curve. This is followed by a fall in arterial pressure and by a simultaneous increase in rate and decrease in amplitude. These are all manifestations of decreased venous return and of decreased stroke volume. After 6–7 seconds a return elevation in pressure can be seen, even though the pressure-squeeze is maintained. This results in the "valley" that is characteristic of the pressure-squeeze curve. The return to higher pressure is the result of a reflex action, which had caused a rise in peripheral resistance in order to prevent a complete disappearance of the blood pressure.

At the end of the pressure-squeeze, there is a brief fall in pressure which is the negative mirror image of the initial pressure peak, and which is the result of the sudden decrease in intrathoracic pressure. After 3 to 4 seconds, the blood pressure again rises and, surprisingly, may exceed the initial pressure peak. This, the so-called "*post-squeeze pressure overshoot*," is due to the rapidly in-

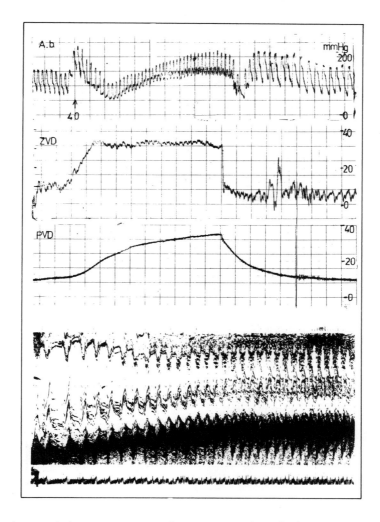

FIG 2–7.

Blood pressure changes during a pressure-exercise (Valsalva). The *upper part* of the figure shows the pressure curves. The top line is arterial pressure that is described in detail in the text. At the 40 mark the subject pushes against a standpipe with a pressure of 40 mm Hg. The middle tracing represents the central venous pressure that reflects the intrathoracic pressure. It shows the sudden rise at the onset of the exercise and the sudden drop at its end. The *lower tracing* represents peripheral venous pressure. The pressure rises slowly as a consequence of the increased intrathoracic pressure and decreased venous return. This slow rise also reflects increasing sympathetic tone and increasing venous wall tension. The *lower part* of the figure represents an echocardiogram during the exercise. The decreasing size of the left ventricle is very noticeable. At the end of the pressure exercise, the septum and posterior wall appear to be in contact.

creasing venous return from the periphery, which leads to an increase in cardiac output, which in turn has to be pumped out against a still elevated peripheral resistance. The consequence of this pressure overshoot is a marked vagal stimulation, via the baroreceptors in the great vessels, which in turn leads to a *postsqueeze bradycardia*. This vagal activity can result in arrhythmias. Even in the healthy person a functional atrioventricular (AV) block or extrasystoles may ap-

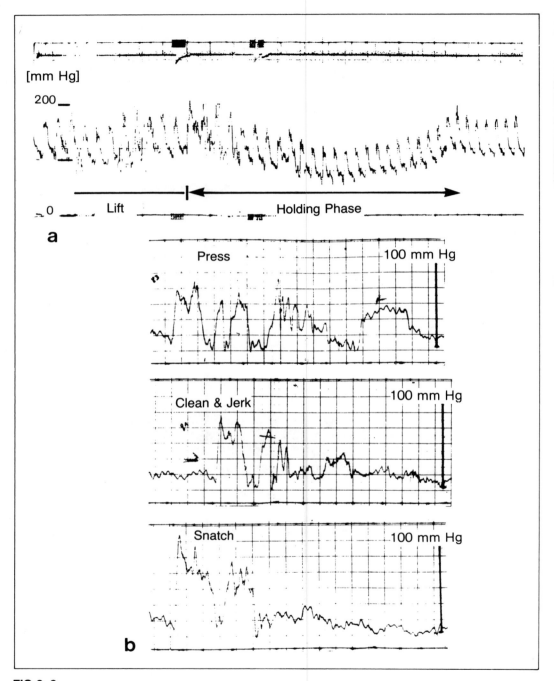

FIG 2–8.

Arterial and central venous pressure during weight lifting. **a,** the arterial pressure curve shows the typical "valley" that is characteristic of the Valsalva maneuver (see Fig 2–7). **b,** central venous pressure measured by telemetry during the three classic forms of weight lifting. It shows a rise of more than 100 mm Hg.

pear and this may be markedly accentuated in the coronary patient. Taking all these events into consideration, it is evident that during the pressure-squeeze exercise, there are a number of danger periods. This does not mean, however, that the pressure-squeeze exercise itself presents a major danger to circulation. In the healthy person it is tolerated without any problems. During the conditioning of the person with a potential circulatory risk, the following considerations must be kept in mind:

1. There are dangerous pressure peaks that may lead to the rupture of some peripheral vessels. In a hypertensive patient this may mean that a resting pressure of 200/100 mm Hg may shoot up to 300/200 mm Hg under the superimposed pressure of the pressure-squeeze exercise. It is obvious that this can lead to an intracranial hemorrhage.

2. The decrease of the cardiac output by 50% also means that the coronary blood flow will decrease by the same amount, as was shown by Benchimol (1972). This raises the risk of myocardial complications, e.g., rhythm disturbances and infarction (see section on "Traumatic Cardiac Injury").

3. The brief hypotensive phase, after the termination of the pressure-squeeze exercise, in combination with the maximal pressure effort, may occasionally lead to syncope, even in the healthy person.

4. Rhythm disturbances may also ensue from the vagal stimulation, in the framework of the post-pressure bradycardia. Extrasystoles may lead at this time to ventricular fibrillation.

5. Venous stasis can lead to perivascular hemorrhage during the pressure phase, particularly in the cerebral region. Cerebral venous pressure and cerebrospinal fluid (CSF) pressure rise in parallel with the rise in peripheral venous pressure.

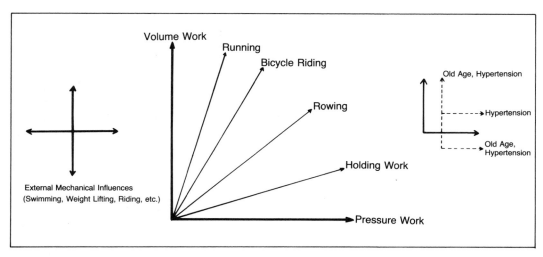

FIG 2–9.

Diagrammatic representation of the behavior of the circulatory volume work and pressure work during different forms of load (exercise). The diagram demonstrates the relative effect of the two types of work. If the *dynamic* part is dominant, the volume work of the circulation increases. When the force (tension) component is in the foreground the increase in blood pressure predominates. These relationships can be modified by endogenous factors *(right)* and external mechanical factors *(left)*. For details, see the text.

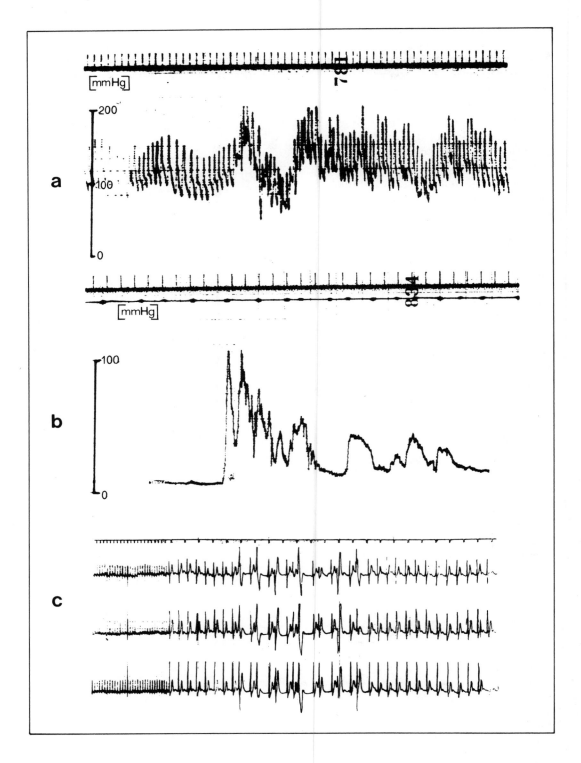

All these findings should provide sufficient grounds to avoid the imposition of maximal pressure-stress on patients with cardiocirculatory disease.

SUMMARY AND CONCLUSION

The previous discussion has shown that under different exercise conditions, the circulatory responses could be different but still followed certain basic rules. In conclusion, we will attempt to bring the different rules into a unified scheme that will allow us to predict the circulatory response, depending on the type of exercise.

This will be attempted in Figure 2–9. The circulatory response is a function of the relative shortening versus tension of the musculature. If the tension of muscle is predominant, pressure-work will be in the foreground. The more pronounced the rhythmic shortening of the muscle, the more prominent the volume-work. This framework will be distorted by a variety of endogenous and exogenous influences. Under external influences we should think primarily about the superimposition of pressure that can displace the indicated coordinates. Such superimposed forces as the hydrostatic pressure in swimming, or the pressure-squeeze force of the Valsalva maneuver, are illustrative. The effects of external pressure are not necessarily only elevations in blood pressure. Negative pressure effects also occur in athletics, e.g., in high jumps from a diving tower and parachute jump-ing. Muscles can also function as an external pressure force, e.g., in wrestling.

The endogenous factors that may affect the relationship between pressure-work and volume-work include physiologic, psychologic, and pathologic factors. As indicated in the discussion about the relationships between age and circulatory responses, in old age there is a shift from volume-work toward pressure-work due to vascular sclerosis. The characteristic psychologic tensions, inherent in athletic events, are the basis for the psychologic increases in pressure-work. Figure 2–10 shows a marked increase in blood pressure, measured in a spectator during the soccer world championship match. This is clearly the result of psychologic tension.

A typical example of the displacement of the pressure-work diagram, due to pathologic causes, can be seen in the reaction pattern of the hypertensive patient. As shown in Figure 2–5, the same intensity of stress causes a higher blood pressure in the hypertensive patient. This may be related, within the framework of atherosclerosis, to a diminished cardiac output. The studies of Julius (1971) have shown, however, that the cardiac output may remain the same or may even rise under similar stress. The ratio of tension-work versus volume-work, and the external and personal factors, allow us to make reasonably accurate predictions about the circulatory responses that can be expected on the basis of the type of stress that is imposed.

FIG 2–10.
Responses in a spectator during an exciting athletic event. **a,** arterial pressure curve in a spectator during a soccer match in which the German national team was competing for the world championship. The segment shown was taken at the time that the German team scored a goal. The arterial pressure rises to 200 mm Hg. The wave form is typical of that seen during the Valsalva maneuver (see Figs 2–7 and 2–8). It was occasioned by the jumping up and yelling, "Goal!" by the spectator. **b,** proves the presence of the Valsalva mechanism: the telemetrically determined central venous pressure rises by more than 100 mm Hg. **c,** shows how such exciting circumstances can lead to arrhythmias. The tracing is taken from a postinfarct patient during the final game for the championship between Germany and The Netherlands in 1974. The patient responded to the winning German goal (2–1) with multifocal premature beats.

3

The Athlete's Heart

> . . . In the final analysis it comes down to this: an enlarged heart is a good thing, if it can perform more work over an extended period of time.
>
> Henschen, 1899
>
> . . . That such a hypertrophy . . . carries in itself the seeds of subsequent insufficiency, is evident, and can be proven by experience, which shows that the majority of professional athletes does not reach old age.
>
> Bruns, 1928

HISTORIC OVERVIEW AND EVALUATION

The athlete's heart is surely one of the oldest and most stimulating subjects for research in sports medicine. The effects of physical activity on the heart were first shown in animals in the last decades of the last century. Bergmann (1884) and Parrot (1893) noted that relative to their body weight, wild animals had much larger hearts, than their domesticated counterparts, e.g., the wild rabbit and the domestic rabbit, etc. Külbs (1906) demonstrated at the beginning of this century that dogs that were made to perform on a treadmill developed cardiac hypertrophy and dilatation under the stimulus of physical activity.

The credit for having described the athlete's heart for the first time in man belongs to Henschen (1899), who published two papers on this subject in the late 19th century. The recognition of the athlete's heart and the development of modern, high-performance athletics are more than coincidence. It should be remembered that the first modern Olympic games were held in 1896. Only competitive sports lead to the development of the athlete's heart, by virtue of the training that they require. Other physical activities, even occupation-related ones, will not do this, even though this has been claimed repeatedly. The concept that this is truly an "athlete's heart," as claimed already by Henschen, is valid. Ever since he coined the phrase "big hearts win races," no other concept has become as well known in sports-medicine than has the athlete's heart.

On the other hand, in the long history of research there has never been as much controversy on any subject than on the interpretation of the athlete's heart. The assessment of the athlete's heart was always a scientific tug-of-war between those who viewed it as a physiologically adapted, extremely effective, and healthy heart, and those who regarded it as sick heart or, at least, a heart at the borderline of the pathologic.

Henschen (1899) arrived at his findings through simple physical diagnostic techniques. The size of the heart was determined through carefully performed percussion. When we consider the later, mistaken interpretations of the athlete's heart made by authors who had much more sophisticated tools at their command, it may be worthwhile to quote the fundamental findings of Henschen, still valid today:

> It follows from this, that skiing causes an enlargement of the heart, and that this enlarged heart can perform more work than the normal heart. There is therefore, a physiologic enlargement of the heart, due to athletic activity: *the athlete's heart.*

Henschen, using his fingers and his mind, came to the conclusion that the athletic enlargement of the heart was based on both dilatation and hypertrophy, or, in modern terminology, on *eccentric hypertrophy.* He wrote further that skiing caused the heart to dilate, particularly in young people, and that later the thickness of this dilated wall increased when the heart had to perform more work. He also observed that all parts of the heart were enlarged and not only the left side. He further found that in the champions both the right and the left side of the heart were enlarged. This symmetrical enlargement is one of the distinctive differences between the athlete's heart and the heart that is enlarged for pathologic reasons, which usually cause only regional enlargement, e.g., aortic valvular stenosis causes an enlargement of the left ventricle and mitral stenosis causes an enlargement of the right ventricle.

This review seems useful in emphasizing the fact that the results of scientific investigation are not necessarily a function of sophisticated instrumentation. I am not suggesting, however, that because of the work of Henschen everything is known about the athlete's heart and that no further investigation and discussion is needed. The introduction of radiologic techniques to determine heart size in athlete's heart studies, accomplished primarily by Scandinavian scientists like Kjellberg (1949), and the reestablishment of the relationship between heart size and performance by Reindell (1954), have given a new impetus to this work. While further discussions about the athlete's heart after the introduction of these techniques seemed pointless, it was again revived when new experimental techniques, such as echocardiography and computed tomography (CT) scanning were introduced in the early 1970s, to give athlete's heart research a new impetus.

The limited techniques available to Henschen naturally also led to some misconceptions. Thus, he described an acute dilatation of the heart after exhausting effort, which to him signaled cardiac failure. Roentgenologic studies performed on athletes a few years later by Moritz (1902), did not substantiate the above findings. The same was true for a number of other investigations that are summarized by Liljestrand (1938).

In spite of the better diagnostic techniques available to him, Moritz (1934) refused to accept the athletic dilatation of the heart as a purely physiologic phenomenon. He tried to equate this type of cardiac enlargement with his ideas of dilatation of the heart as the result of acute strain (tonogenic dilatation) or as the result of acute myocardial failure (myogenic dilatation). In a study done jointly with Dietlen (1908), he expressed a fear that the continued and excessive strain on the heart could lead to an early collapse of the cardiovascular system.

Even this brief review of the "childhood" of the athlete's heart indicates the controversial assessment that runs like a red thread through its almost century-long history. A few examples should show that the interpretation of Henschen that the athlete's heart was well within the physiologic limits was by no means accepted by others.

Deutsch (1924) defined the enlargement of the trained heart as being based on a preexisting weakness. Kaufmann (1933) considered it as the result of a constitutional deficiency. Lysholm (1934) explained the development of the athlete's heart on the basis of the Starling principle, i.e., dilatation, on the basis of overexertion. The fear that such an enlargement of the heart carried the germ of a later insufficiency was expressed by Bruns, as part of an address at the Congress of German Sports Physicians in 1928. It is quoted at the beginning of this section. Bruns expressed that opinion, which seemed entirely natural to him, since it represented a century-old view on the effects of athletics on the cardiocirculatory system, namely, that athletes did not grow old. This view was particularly widely held in the Anglo-American literature of the 19th century, as shown in the review of this subject by Roskamm (1964). The life-expectancy of the athlete was believed to be shortened, in spite of the epidemiologic studies that did not support this view and that are reviewed in the same publication. The epidemiologic studies show that there is no relationship between the athlete's heart and *life expectancy*. The athlete's heart is a highly effective heart, but its owner lives neither shorter, as previously believed, nor longer, than the average of the population.

This change of mind concerning the effects of athletics on the "durability" of the cardiovascular system can be illustrated with another quotation. While it is generally accepted today that physical activity is an important factor in the prevention of atherosclerosis, the following quotation can be found in the work of Luda in a listing of the risk factors important in the development of sclerotic vascular changes: "There is no question but that the currently very common excessive athletic efforts are a frequent cause of arteriosclerosis . . . almost all professional athletes, sooner or later develop such injuries, due to overexertion."

Such erroneous interpretations are by no means limited to the older literature. The most surprising interpretation can be found in the standard American cardiology textbook by Friedberg (1972), which, even in a new edition, over ten years ago made the statement that while the athlete's heart was formerly considered to be a physiologic adaptation, it is today interpreted as a result of overexertion in a rheumatic, syphilitic, or congenitally damaged heart.

The old misgivings concerning the athlete's heart are cast into new forms in the recent literature and are supported by new arguments. In a review of the problems of sudden cardiac death, Keren (1981) concludes that such sudden death was more common among athletes. According to his opinion, this seems to be the result of the changes that are subsumed under the heading of athlete's heart. The author bases this opinion on the likelihood of more frequent cardiac arrhythmias among athletes. This view is totally unsupported by epidemiologic studies.

Rhythm changes in athletes are most frequently found in the form of bradycardias. The "training-bradycardia" in athletes trained for endurance can result in heart rates of 30 beats per minute. It can be asked, and frequently is asked in practice, whether physical conditioning does not necessarily lead to a future requirement for an artificial pacemaker. Franz (1979) reported the case of a long distance runner whose heart rate became consecutively less and less, until finally a complete heart block required electrical pacing. An interesting new concern about the athlete's heart was developed from an observation of Maron (1980). He could demonstrate a hypertrophic cardiomyopathy in 14 of 29 athletes who died suddenly. The studies of Morganroth (1975) showed that the heart of high performance athletes frequently showed a thickening of the septum, similar to that found in patients with an asymmetrical septal hypertrophy.

This raises the question whether the physiologic hypertrophy can indeed lead to pathologic changes. This then brings us right back to where we started from. It comes back to the old defensive attitude concerning unlimited physical exercise and the athletic cardiac enlargement that arose from the above quoted studies. It is now raised to a new and higher level of discussion. All these suspicions about the athlete's heart can be gathered together under the term *athlete's heart syndrome* that appears particularly frequently in the American literature. A medical dictionary defines the term syndrome as "a group of symptoms that appear at the same time."

The frequent interpretation of the athlete's heart as a sick organ is readily understandable. The physiologist observes an enlargement of the heart in his experimental animals as the result of overexertion. The clinician views the enlargement of the heart as an indication of incipient failure. For him, an increasing heart size is always a negative diagnostic sign. To this has to be added that the enlarged athlete's heart is frequently accompanied by other changes, particularly electrocardiographic (ECG) abnormalities. The false assumption that claims that "a large heart is a sick heart" when applied to the athlete's heart is based on the lack of recognition that in physiologic experiments the adaptation factor of cardiac enlargement is missing. The clinician fails to recognize the fact that in the athlete the enlargement of the heart also denotes an improvement in performance.

In order to explain this relationship between cardiac enlargement and increased efficiency Reindell (1960) introduced the concept of *regulatory cardiac enlargement*. This is in contrast to the tonogenic and myogenic cardiac dilation described by Moritz. Reindell also systematically quantified the relationship between cardiac size and performance as a criterion of the adaptive response. This will be discussed in detail below. An im-

portant argument in favor of the value of the athlete's heart as an adaptation phenomenon was developed through intracardiac pressure measurements, at rest and under stress, by Kindermann, Knipping, Musshoff, and Reindell, who were unable to show any pathologic flow-pressure relationships. In further discussions concerning the athlete's heart, increasing emphasis was placed on the positive value of this condition from a general health point of view. This was based on the functional economy of the process, which allowed performance of an equal effort at significantly lower heart rates. This modus operandi, with its sparing effect on cardiac oxygen requirements, has become a model that has been used to highlight the usefulness of physical conditioning in the management of cardiac patients. This was already emphasized by Ewig in 1932.

Even if in isolated cases the above suspicions may be justified and exercise may aggravate a preexisting pathologic condition, it must be emphasized most strongly that studies carried out over many years have substantiated the basic premise of Henschen (1899) concerning the athlete's heart, namely that "an enlarged heart is a good thing if it can perform more work over an extended period of time." It could never be proved that the development of the athlete's heart had ever exceeded the physiologic limits. In the following sections the dimensional, functional, and clinical aspects of this remarkable heart will be discussed.

DIMENSIONAL CHANGES

Anatomic Findings

A literature review of the anatomic findings in athlete's heart reveals an impressive lack of data on this subject, other than the studies of Kirch that were published in the 1930s. There are some publications on the findings in athletes who died suddenly, but these authors were more concerned with the cause of death than with the peculiarities of physiologic hypertrophy. For this reason we must still depend for anatomic considerations of the athlete's heart on the findings of Kirch, which are not very satisfactory, since the athletes he examined, according to their history, cannot be considered as having been fully trained. In this regard we must recognize, that both the intensity and the extent of training has increased considerably since the 1930s.

Kirch presented his results in two talks in 1935 and 1936. He had collected data on 35 athletes who died suddenly, either during exercise or at rest. He was personally involved in 14 cases, but had to rely on autopsy findings for the others. There was a marked difference in the athletic activities and in the intensity of training among these athletes.

Kirch's most significant finding was the demonstration that cardiac hypertrophy was the result of physical exercise. This was by no means taken for granted by other pathologists prior to this time. Aschoff (1928) recognized cardiac enlargement as a consequence of general physical conditioning, not as a part of an adaptation mechanism. In contrast Kirch found that in some athletes the heart was twice as large as normal. According to his interpretation, these were healthy hearts that could even reduce the hypertrophy after the physical conditioning had been discontinued. He found no evidence of cardiac damage that could be attributed to physical training.

Another important point emerging from the findings of Kirch, is the fact that the hypertrophy need not always be symmetrical and that preferential enlargement of the right or left heart could be observed. In most cases, though, the right ventricular hypertrophy predominates. Kirch was unable to assign these differences in hypertrophy to any specific athletic activity. The observation that right-sided hypertrophy is dominant is of in-

terest in the context of the high incidence of an incomplete right bundle-branch block in the ECG of athletes, which will be discussed below.

For this reason the concept of the *harmonious hypertrophy* of the athlete's heart, introduced by Linzbach (1958), cannot be applied fully to the symmetrical enlargement of all heart chambers and walls, as it is done frequently. Actually, Linzbach never meant to apply this term in this way. He was trying to establish a global system of the different hypertrophies, which was to include both physiologic as well as pathologic forms. The concept of the "harmonious hypertrophy" was meant to indicate that the microscopic structure of the physiologically hypertrophied muscle was identical to the normal myocardium, but as though looked at "through a magnifying glass." In contrast to the physiologic hypertrophy, the pathologic hypertrophy is characterized by a *structural dilatation* that represents an early state of heart failure. Such a structural dilatation was said to be present, when the limits of the *critical weight* of the heart were exceeded. This critical weight limit was set at 500 gm, a weight never observed by Kirch in the athletes he examined.

When taking into consideration the new histochemical findings (Walpurger, 1970) it becomes possible to extrapolate Linzbach's ideas from the field of microscopy to that of biochemistry. The enzymatic pattern in the trained heart differs only quantitatively, but not qualitatively from the untrained heart.

There is a marked difference here, when compared to the skeletal muscle in which we can find distinct variations, dependent on the type of conditioning. In skeletal muscle we find the so-called slow-contracting or red fibers, which are predominantly characterized by enzymes of the anaerobic metabolism group and which can be found in large numbers only in the athlete trained for endurance. In the musculature of the sprinter or the "power" athlete, we find mostly white fibers, which have few enzymes of the aerobic, energy-liberating type, but many of the anaerobic, energy storage enzymes. The uniformity of work seen in the heart muscle is also manifested in the uniformity of structure. In the skeletal muscle, however, specific kinds of performance require specific muscular structures.

Linzbach (1958) emphasized the fact that the number of the cardiac muscle fibers remained constant in physiologic hypertrophy. This constancy in the number of fibers and the inability of the cardiac muscle to become hyperplastic after birth is, according to Linzbach, not the reason why the critical heart weight is maintained, although this was alleged frequently. Since the muscle cells cannot divide, extreme hypertrophy must lead to an increase in the diffusion path for oxygen to the center of the cell. This raises the danger of a possible central cellular necrosis. According to the findings of Linzbach, the relationship between capillaries and the number of fibers remains constant, even when the critical heart weight is exceeded, a situation in which there may be hyperplasia as well. He saw coronary insufficiency as the cause for the "structural" dilatation and believed that the insufficiency was due to an insufficient development of the coronary vessels and their ostia and to concomitant arteriosclerotic changes and not to an increase in the diameter of the muscle fibers.

Contrary to the views of Linzbach, the possibility of myocardial hyperplasia in humans after birth remained an open question in the literature, even after some animal experiments that made the possibility of such a hyperplasia likely (Kleitke, 1977). There is another matter in the studies of Linzbach and Kirch that must be discussed. This is the absolute value of the *critical heart weight*, as de-

termined by these authors. As already mentioned, the athletes examined by Kirch were only incompletely trained by our present standards and only four of them were professional athletes. Of the well documented cases that he studied himself, the heaviest heart weighed 530 gm and belonged to a professional boxer. According to our own experience, one cannot count on the presence of a significantly enlarged athlete's heart at all in boxers. These athletes never exceed a heart volume of 1,200 ml. It is hardly likely that the heart of a bicycle racer or long distance runner, trained to the point of extreme endurance, and showing cardiac volumes of up to 1,700 ml, should not be heavier than that.

On this basis we can assume that there are athlete's hearts that clearly exceed a weight of 500 gm. It also seems likely that the limits of the critical heart weight cannot be determined precisely, and that they depend on individual factors, e.g., total body size. If 500 gm are really the absolute limit, then, logically, a small athlete should be more trainable than a large one, since the small athlete would reach the critical heart weight only later. The conclusion is inescapable that the critical heart weight cannot be considered as dogma. If, however, we interpret this concept to mean that the physiologic cardiac hypertrophy must have its limits, then this model makes excellent sense. The development of athletics during the last few decades may well emphasize such a concept. Although the dimensions and the intensity of athletic training and the achievements of the athletes have grown enormously since the 1950s, when Reindell (1960) first used radiologic techniques to determine the heart size of athletes, we do not find larger heart sizes in athletes today, using the same radiologic methodology. For this reason it must be assumed that the limits of physiologic cardiac hypertrophy are reached relatively soon, and that further improvements through training must lie in metabolic and peripheral-vascular adaptations.

RADIOLOGIC FINDINGS

After the already-mentioned radiologic studies by Moritz (1902), the next step was the planimetric, quantitative evaluation of the heart size by the same author in 1934. His findings do not, however, reflect our current knowledge of the athlete's heart. He found, for example, no enlargement of the heart in swimmers, who belong to the endurance athletes, while he did observe athlete's hearts in wrestlers, who are usually not trained for endurance to any significant degree. His opinion may have been based on an inherent error in assessing the third dimension, since planimetric studies do not take into account the increase in depth of the heart.

The latter concept was introduced by Scandinavian authors, using *cardiac volume* measurements. Rohrer (1916) was the first one to use this technique that was repeated, independently, by Kahlstorf (1933). These two authors must be given the credit for heart volume determination. Kjellberg (1949) was the first one to show a correlation between achievements and radiologic heart volume. To quantify such a relationship, Nylin (1933) introduced an index, known by his name, that is a ratio of the heart volume and the stroke volume. This index was the first attempt to answer mathematically the original question by Henschen (1899) of whether an enlarged heart can perform greater work.

In view of the technical difficulties in measuring stroke volume routinely, Reindell replaced it in the index with the maximal oxygen uptake per heart beat, the so-called *maximal oxygen pulse*. This index was used widely to differentiate between physiologic and pathologic en-

largement of the heart. In this way Reindell combined the radiologic evaluation of the athlete's heart with the functional considerations obtained by spiro-ergometry under *maximal, in vivo conditions*. This approach was introduced clinically by Knipping and his co-workers and to sports medicine by Hollmann (1959). According to Reindell, an athlete's heart can be considered to be normal if the relationship between heart size and the maximal oxygen pulse lies within normal limits.

Since this approach continues to have practical importance today, it will be presented in some technical detail. The *radiologic determination of heart size* is accomplished today in Germany on the basis of the Rohrer-Kahlstorf formula, as modified by Musshoff (1956). The determination of heart volume is done in the supine position from a focal distance of 2 meters to avoid the orthostatic filling distortions of the heart and to have parallel rays, which allow the assessment of the heart size without distortion. The surface area of the heart is determined on a PA film, on which an oval area is drawn with a length of L and a width of W. To measure the depth (D) a lateral film is taken during a barium swallow. This process is illustrated diagrammatically in Figure 3–1. Considering that the heart is not a rectangular structure, a correction factor becomes necessary. The volume of the heart is than calculated by the following formula:

Heart volume (HV) $= 0.4 \times W \times L \times D$

The *maximal oxygen pulse* is determined by spiro-ergometry during a stress test. It represents the maximal oxygen uptake divided by the maximal achievable heart rate. Assuming that the maximal oxygen uptake in the untrained individual is about 3 L/minute, the maximal oxygen pulse will be approximately 15 ml. In the trained individual who can double his maximal oxygen uptake to 6 L/minute without significantly changing his maximal heart rate, a maximal oxygen pulse of 30 ml can thus be achieved. If one relates this maximal oxygen pulse to the heart volume, rather than to the stroke volume, we get the formula for the *heart volume-performance quotient* (HVPQ):

$$\text{HVPQ} = \frac{\text{Heart volume}}{\text{Maximal oxygen pulse}} =$$

$$\frac{\text{Heart volume}}{\text{Max oxygen uptake} \times \text{max heart rate}^{-1}}$$

The HVPQ is also know as the *heart volume equivalent* value. Assuming a mean cardiac volume of 750 ml, the performance quotient can be calculated to be a dimensionless number of about 50. If the heart becomes larger under the influence of physical training, its performance should rise correspondingly. If, for example, the volume of the heart doubles, to 1500 ml, the maximal oxygen pulse must also double, to abut 30 ml, for the performance quotient to remain the same.

If the heart enlarges under pathologic conditions, its performance does not increase correspondingly and the quotient becomes larger. A quotient of 60 can be regarded as the lower margin of pathologic values.

Naturally, this method provides only a rough screen for the evaluation of cardiac enlargement. Nevertheless, it serves as a good practical guide. The clinician is frequently confronted with the question of whether the cardiac enlargement in a patient who claims to be engaged in athletics indicates a pathologic state, or whether it is the result of physical conditioning. In this situation the establishment of a relationship between physical performance and the degree of enlargement of the heart makes sense. The performance quotient can be estimated, even if spiro-ergometry is not available, if the relationship between mechanical performance and oxygen uptake is known. As

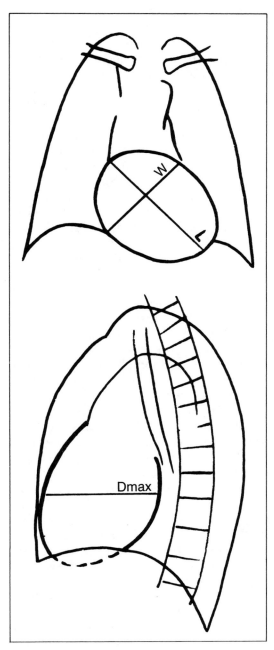

FIG 3–1.
Diagrammatic representation of the determination of heart size by roentgenographic techniques. The heart volume is derived by the product of the length *(L)* and width *(W)* of the oval obtained on a PA view, being multiplied by the greatest depth *(Dmax)* obtained from a lateral view. The product must be multiplied by 0.4, which represents a correction factor.

indicated above, in the discussion of the hemodynamic adaptation reaction, the increase in oxygen utilization is approximately 12 ml/min for each watt performance. The oxygen uptake for any given intensity of stress is:

$$VO_2 = 300 + 12 \times \text{performance (in watts) (ml/min)}$$

The number 300 in the equation represents the resting oxygen uptake. If, for example, a patient whose heart volume has increased to 1,200 ml can achieve a maximal 200 watts at a pulse rate of 180 in an ergometric test, it can be calculated that he will have a maximum oxygen uptake of 2.7 L/minute and a maximal oxygen pulse of 15 ml. The HVPQ is a pathologic 80; the physical performance potential does not correspond to the increased size of the heart.

Modern hospitals naturally have additional diagnostic procedures available for the functional evaluation of the heart. These can be used in doubtful cases and include echocardiography, Swann-Ganz catheterization, etc. Establishing the relationship between the size of the heart and its performance limits is important, since it will always show that the frequently made clinical error, which declares that an athlete's heart is a sick heart purely on the basis of its size, is improper, if simultaneous consideration is not given to its performance.

An error in the opposite direction, which is also frequently seen, is to declare that the enlargement of the heart is due to physical training, even though the size of the heart and its capacity for performance are not in proper relationship. This error can also be avoided by the above considerations. It must be emphasized at this time that the amount of physical exercise necessary for the development of an athlete's heart is usually underestimated. Only the training that leads to high performance athletics with an endurance component can result in an athlete's heart. Mass athletic activity or occupational activity are never sufficient to produce an increase in heart size. In addition, the physiologic hypertrophy quickly regresses once the training stimulus stops. Physical activity in youth cannot be the basis on which to declare that an enlarged heart in an older person is an "athlete's heart" when this person has not engaged in athletics for several decades. When evaluating cardiac enlargement in the athlete by radiologic means, it must be remembered that the enlargement is less evident in the PA view and in the standing position. This view usually indicates only a slight enlargement or a heart at the upper limits of normal, which could have an aortic or mitral configuration. The true extent of the cardiac enlargement can be determined only by measuring the cardiac volume (Fig 3–2). When evaluating the cardiac volume, it must be remembered that the volume, in principle, depends on two factors: the total mass of the body and the functional capacity of the heart. The weight lifter also has an enlarged heart, but this enlargement is in relation to the body mass. In contrast to this, the heart of the athlete trained for endurance also enlarges in relationship to body weight. This becomes evident by looking at the cardiac volume data obtained in the Cologne Institute for Circulatory Research and Sportsmedicine in champion athletes (Fig 3–3). In these athletes, there is very good correlation between heart size and oxygen uptake.

The average, weight-related cardiac volume in the male is about 11 ml/kg body weight, i.e., approximately 825 ml in a 75-kg man. The values in the female are smaller both in absolute terms and also in their relationship to weight. They are approximately 10 ml/kg body weight. The upper limits of normal are 12 ml/kg for the male and 11 ml/kg in the female.

The absolute largest athlete's heart was found to be 1,700 ml. This was

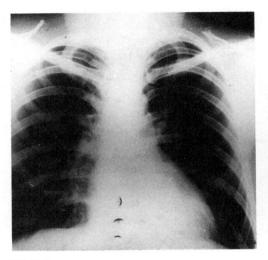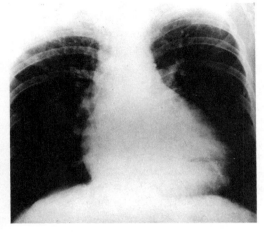

FIG 3–2.
Left, the heart of the best-known postwar bicycle racer in the PA view. **Right,** the same heart in the supine position, taken to determine the cardiac volume.

found in a water polo player by Medved (1964) and in a bicycle racer by Hollmann (1965). Both forms of athletics have one thing in common, i.e., that the body mass is of little significance, since it is supported by the very nature of the activity, water in one instance and the bicycle in the other. This also explained why the heart of the runner never reaches the same absolute value. Relative to body

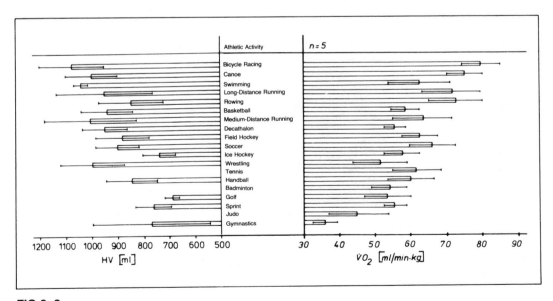

FIG 3–3.
The maximal cardiac volumes *(left)* and maximal average O_2 uptake values obtained from the five best athletes of different athletic disciplines ever studied in the Cologne Institute for Circulatory Research and Sports-Medicine. The largest hearts and largest O_2 uptake values were seen in endurance athletes. The two values correlated very well (after Heck, quoted after Hollmann).

mass, however, very high values are found in the long distance runners. The highest value ever described was found by Reindell. It was 20.8 ml/kg body weight (Keul, 1982).

The largest heart found in a female athlete, 1,150 ml, was reported by Medved in a cross-country skier. Relative to weight, this heart was also smaller (16.0 ml/kg) than the hearts of the male champion athletes. This observation underlines the fact that physiologic cardiac hypertrophy is both absolutely and relatively smaller in the female than in the male. This matter should probably remain open and may have to be revised later as more and more women participate in intensive endurance training, in accordance with the spirit of the times.

The Electrocardiographic Signs of Hypertrophy

A characteristic ECG of a hypertrophic athlete's heart is shown in Figure 3–4. In contrast to radiologic techniques, the ECG has not proved to be a very useful noninvasive diagnostic aid in athlete's heart hypertrophy. There is general agreement in the literature that the ECG parameters of left- and right-ventricular hypertrophy in the athlete bear little relationship to the anatomic findings. The overlap between the endurance-trained and untrained person is considerable. The literature will not be reviewed here, since the ECG peculiarities have been the subject of an earlier publication (Rost, 1980). The modest predictive value of the *Sokolow-Lyon index* for left ventricular

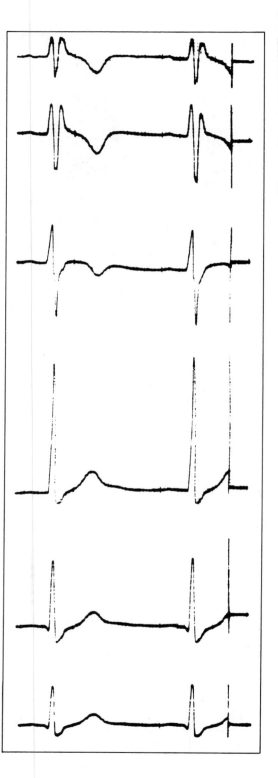

FIG 3–4.
Typical signs of hypertrophy in the athlete's heart electrocardiogram. Right-sided hypertrophy is shown by the right sided delay in the form of an "M" shaped ventricular complex in leads V_1 and V_2. The left-sided hypertrophy is manifested in the very high R wave in lead V_4.

hypertrophy can be seen in Figure 3–5, where the minimally endurance-trained ball players show the highest indices. Table 3–1 shows the low, nonsignificant correlation between the heart volume and the Sokolow-Lyon index on the one hand and the echocardiographic findings and ECG criteria on the other.

It can be concluded from these observations that although an elevation of the Sokolow-Lyon index can frequently be found in the athlete, this is, as a rule, an indication of particularly good conductivity in the young, well-trained athlete and not a sign of cardiac hypertrophy. This fact must be taken into consideration before the athlete is diagnosed as a cardiac patient, which happens only too frequently. If the radiologic findings and the echocardiogram do not indicate a significant hypertrophy, the ECG findings should be accordingly qualified.

As far as the ECG representation of the athlete's heart hypertrophy is concerned, Schmidt (1961) suggests that this should be looked at as the expression of an ideal *double-volume hypertrophy*, since all areas of the heart are more or less involved in the hypertrophy. This means that with all chambers symmetrically enlarged, the ECG should be generally unchanged. On the other hand, the already-discussed findings of Kirch (1935, 1936) suggest that there may be a

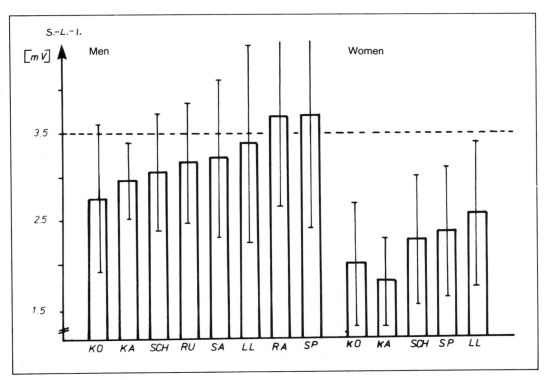

FIG 3–5.

Left ventricular Sokolow-Lyon index in male and female athletes in our study group collected by Reinke (1982). *KO*, control group; *KA*, canoe paddlers; *Sch*, swimmers; *RV*, oarsmen; *SA*, heavy athletes; *LL*, long distance runner; *RA*, bicycle racer; *SP*, team sport player. The normal upper limit of the left ventricular Sokolow-Lyon index of 3.5 mV is indicated by the broken line. It is exceeded by a number of athletes as indicated by the standard deviations. There appears to be no relationship to endurance training. The team sport players who are relatively poorly trained for endurance show the highest values for this index.

TABLE 3–1.

Relationships Observed Between Echocardiographic, Roentgenologic, and ECG Criteria in Evaluation of Left Ventricular Hypertrophy in Athletes

PARAMETERS*		DEGREE OF REGRESSION	R	P
y:RV$_5$ + SV$_1$	♂	y = 0.0009; x + 2.49	.20	.033
x:HV	♀	y = 0.0011; x + 1.40	.24	.053
	♂ ♀	y = 0.0024; x + 0.90	.45	≤.001
y:RV$_5$ + SV$_1$	♂	y = .3687; x + .520	.27	.003
x:TED	♀	y = −.2911; x + 4.112	−.06	.651
	♂ ♀	y = .5784; x − 1.326	.41	≤.001
y:HV	♂	y = 245.0; x − 399.1	.70	≤.001
x:LVID$_d$	♀	y = 117.7; x + 81.9	.58	≤.001
	♂ ♀	y = 284.7; x − 662.6	.75	≤.001
y:HV	♂	y = 661.9; x + 262.0	.53	≤.001
x:LVWD$_d$	♀	y = 164.1; x + 517.3	.26	≤.036
	♂ ♀	y = 865.9; x − 9.4	.64	≤.001
y:HV	♂	y = 189.5; x − 491.8	.75	≤.001
x:TED	♀	x = 101.1; x − 18.7	.60	≤.001
	♂ ♀	y = 220.3; x − 761.3	.81	≤.001

*Left ventricular Sokolow-Lyon Index = RV$_5$ + SV$_1$; cardiac volume = HV; total echocardiographic, left ventricular diameter (TED) = sum of left ventricular internal diameter at the end of *systole* (LVID$_d$) plus left ventricular wall thickness in diastole (LVWD$_d$) plus the thickness of the septum. The correlations show that there is a poor relationship between the cardiac volume and Sokolow-Lyon index, but that there was a good correlation between the echocardiographic and roentgenologic parameters (after Reinke, 1982).

predominance of right ventricular hypertrophy. It seems possible that the relatively frequently encountered *right-sided conduction delay* and *incomplete right bundle-branch block* may be explained in athletes on the basis of this slight right-sided hypertrophy (see Fig 3–4).

A review of the literature and a reference to the ECG monograph reveals that depending on the author, 10% to 50% of all athletes demonstrate an incomplete right bundle-branch block. When the right precordial lead tracings are included, this number rises to 80% and if the vector cardiographic findings are also included, the incidence is 90%. The interpretation of an incomplete right bundle-branch block as a consequence of physical training is by no means unanimous and is questioned by Butschenko (1966) among others. On the other hand,

Roskamm (1966) found a clear correlation between cardiac hypertrophy and the relative frequency of incomplete right bundle-branch block. Roskamm also found a regression of this finding upon discontinuation of the training.

On the basis of these findings it would seem that the right-sided delay in conduction is well documented in the athlete as an expression of a physiologic hypertrophy. It should be emphasized, for the sake of the medical practice, that the concept of the incomplete right bundle-branch block is a singularly unfortunate one because the ECG, which shows these changes, in no way represents a "block." Unfortunately, it can be seen again and again that the athlete who is told that he has a "heart block" is made unnecessarily anxious. For this reason the "block" concept should be avoided in connection with the athlete's heart ECG. It would be better to use a purely descriptive term such as physiologic right-sided delay, or M-shaped chamber complex in V_1, rSR, etc.

ECHOCARDIOGRAPHIC FINDINGS

Although the discussions concerning the anatomy of the athlete's heart seemed to be closed with the autopsy findings of Kirch (1935, 1936) and the radiologic findings of Reindell, in the closing years of the 1950s a strong new impulse was given to these discussions by the introduction of ultrasound imaging. Sports medicine and ultrasound seem to have been created for each other. On the one hand, the athlete is the ideal candidate for echocardiographic studies, by virtue of an absence of pulmonary emphysema, a thin layer of fat, and an enlarged heart. On the other hand sports medicine must rely primarily on noninvasive diagnostic techniques. Yet, to date the echocardiogram has not been able to replace the radiogram entirely, since even the two-dimensional "sector-scan" cannot give a complete representation of the heart.

Ultrasound compensates for one of the significant shortcomings of routine radiography, i.e., the inability to distinguish between the chamber of the heart and the wall of the heart. The echocardiogram makes it possible to investigate one of the old arguments about the athlete's heart, i.e., the distinction between dilatation and hypertrophy. In addition, echocardiography opens new possibilities in evaluating the function of the athlete's heart and also in diagnostics that will be further discussed later.

In view of these advantages, it is understandable that in the last decade a large number of studies have been performed in this area since we first published echocardiographic findings in athletes at the time of the Olympic games in Munich (Rost, 1972). This literature can also not be fully discussed and the interested reader is referred to a detailed monograph for further information (Rost, 1982). As shown in a typical example (Fig 3–6) and in mean values obtained from about 500 athletes (Fig 3–7), the dilatation of the chambers and the thickening of the wall can be demonstrated extremely well.

A new perspective on athlete's heart was introduced on echocardiographic grounds by Morganroth (1975, 1977) who was the first one to emphasize that there may be a very particular form of cardiac adaptation in power athletes, a fact previously totally denied. The athlete's heart was believed to belong entirely to the endurance-trained athlete. Morganroth found a "pure (concentric) hypertrophy" in power athletes, as contrasted with the "pure dilatation" in the endurance athlete. Such a response model seems perfectly understandable when one considers the different hemodynamic conditions that prevail in the primarily dynamic-isotonic work as compared with the predominantly isometric work. In the first case the volume-work stands in the foreground, in the second case the pressure-work stands in the foreground.

Yet, on purely theoretical grounds the simple distinction made by Morganroth cannot be correct. It is contradicted by other findings, including our own (see Fig 3–7). According to Laplace's law, an enlargement of the inner space of the heart must be accompanied by an increase in wall tension. A dilatation must therefore always be accompanied by a thickening of the wall to compensate for the work of the individual muscle fiber. As discussed earlier, Henschen has stated that there had to be a simultaneous hypertrophy and dilatation, even in the endurance trained athlete. Figure 3–7 shows that larger hearts have thicker walls, even if they belong to endurance athletes. This is in contrast to the find-

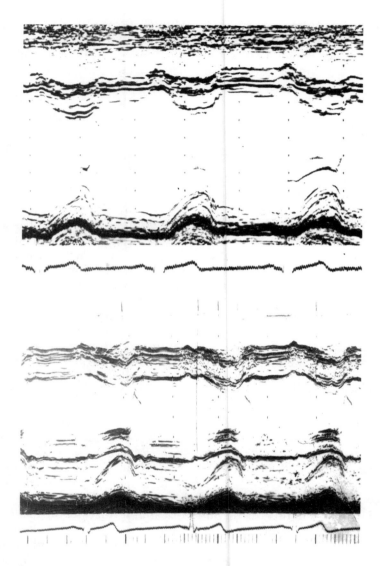

FIG 3–6.
Comparison of typical echocardiograms in an endurance athlete *(top)* and a power athlete *(bottom)*. The echocardiogram of the endurance athlete belongs to the world champion professional bicycle racer. It is notable for the end-diastolic left ventricular diameter of 70 mm. The wall is only moderately thickened. The echocardiogram of the power athlete belongs to a well-known German weight lifting champion. The left ventricular diameter of 53 mm is only minimally increased, but there is definite thickening of the walls and particularly of the septum.

ings of Morganroth. The cardiac enlargement of the endurance-trained athlete is, therefore, not pure dilatation but an *eccentric hypertrophy*.

The findings of Morganroth in power athletes seem unlikely. He found an essentially normal left ventricular diameter and a considerable thickening of the ventricular wall, i.e., concentric hypertrophy in a world-class shot-putter, whose body was huge as indicated by a body surface of 2.52 m². As known from radiologic findings, the cardiac size should increase in parallel with the increase in body size,

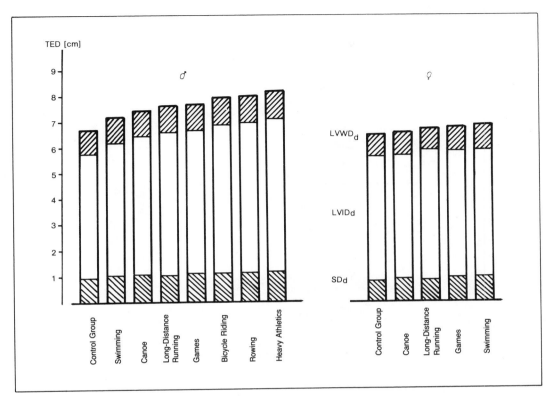

FIG 3–7.
Echocardiographic measurements in different male and female athletic groups from our own investigations (collected by Reinke, 1982). $LVWD_d$, left ventricular wall thickness; $LVID_d$, left ventricular internal diameter; SD_d, septum thickness; *TED,* total end-diastolic diameter as the sum of the internal diameter, wall and septal thickness.

so that in this person a greater-than-average left ventricular diameter would have been expected. Our findings, given in Figure 3–7, support this expectation.

Although the conception of Morganroth in itself is too simplistic, it may have some validity in a modified form. According to other findings both endurance-sports and power-sports lead to cardiac hypertrophy. Dilatation predominates in the endurance athlete and hypertrophy in the power athlete (Simon, 1981) (Fig 3–8).

This subject is very difficult to discuss, since even a normal increase in body mass has an effect on the relationship of wall thickness to diameter. When considering that the body size of the power athlete is usually well above the general average, it is difficult to determine whether the myocardial hypertrophy is due to the power sport or to the body size. In spite of these problems, the findings of Simon seem to show clearly that power athletes do have a hypertrophy. These findings were substantiated by Longhurst (1980). This author found the same cardiac diameter in weight lifters as in nonathletes of equal body surface, although the weight lifters had thicker cardiac walls and septa. When the left ventricular muscle mass, as determined by echocardiography is placed in relationship with the skeletal muscle mass, the results are not different in the nontrained person. In contrast, it was found that in the endurance athlete there

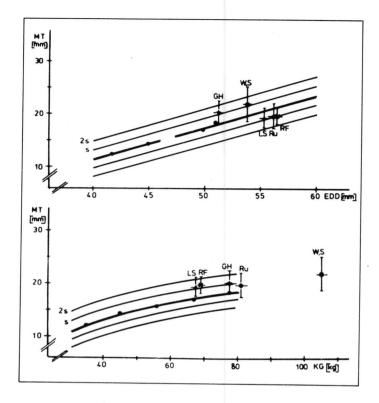

FIG 3–8.
The relationship between the total left ventricular wall thickness (*MT* = sum of the left ventricular wall thickness and the septal thickness) and the end-diastolic ventricular diameter *(EDD)* and body weight *(KG)* (after Simon 1981). The correlation coefficients and scatter show normal values. The following groups are represented: power athletes *(GH, weight lifters; WS,* throwers-shot putters) and endurance athletes *(LS, long distance runners; RF, bicycle riders; RV, rowers).* Both groups show an increase in wall thickness in relation to body weight when compared to the nontrained person. In relationship to the left ventricular diameter, the wall thickness is high in the power athletes and low in the endurance athlete.

was an increased cardiac muscle mass, even in relationship to weight. According to these findings, isometric training leads to a hypertrophy of the left ventricular muscle mass in parallel to the total body muscle mass. According to Dickhuth (1979), this hypertrophy is particularly marked in the septum.

Our findings did not fully substantiate the above observations, even though we also found some weight lifters who had thickened cardiac walls (see Fig 3–6). Similar echos could be found also in the endurance trained athletes (see Fig 3–10). In athletes, we found a ratio of 1:1 between the septum and the thickness of the posterior wall. The ratio of the heart wall thickness to ventricular diameter was 1:5.5 without clear differences between athletes from different athletic disciplines or between athletes and nonathletes.

Such differences in the literature must be explained on the ground of differences in methodology. It is difficult to determine cardiac hypertrophy through "single beam" measurement, as is done with the M-mode technique. As discussed in the section on "Heart Volume," we consider the likelihood of calculating the left ventricular muscle mass from M-mode echo as highly doubtful.

The differences in myocardial wall thickness found in athletes is quite small. While the left ventricular diameter can increase from 5 cm in the nontrained person to 5.5 to 6 cm, or in extraordinary cases even to 7 cm in the trained person, the thickness of the myocardial wall will increase only by 1–2 mm. The thickness of the wall cannot always be measured accurately and the measurement of the right ventricular septum is particularly unreliable (Fig 3–9). Consequently it will have to remain an open question if a sports-specific hypertrophy exists in the power athlete. The question is if the elevation in blood pressure in the power

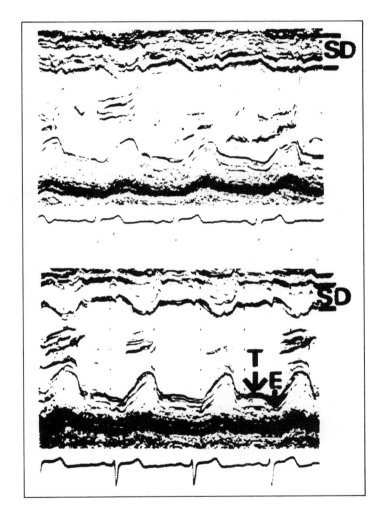

FIG 3–9.

These echocardiograms were obtained from a weight lifter. The upper echo seems to show a definite increase in septum thickness *(SD)* and posterior wall thickness. This is probably due, however, to lack of clear definition of the right and left endocardial borders. When the sensitivity of the imaging was changed, it appears that the right ventricular area was probably obscured by the superposition of a trabecular muscle. The septum is in fact thinner than had been assumed previously. The same is true for the posterior wall, where a trabecular muscle echo *(T)* simulates a true endocardial echo *(E)*. This example illustrates the possibility of serious echocardiographic errors in the interpretation of the athlete's heart.

athlete, of short duration when calculated on a 24-hour basis is sufficient to produce hypertrophy. Studies performed by our group (Reinke, 1982) in young, hypertensive patients, in whom the median 24-hour pressure is surely higher, showed no clear-cut hypertrophy. The solution to this problem will have to wait until the two-dimensional echocardiography is developed to the point to where it is possible to define the entire left ventricular endocardium without any difficulty (Fig 3–10).

DEVELOPMENT AND REGRESSION OF THE ATHLETE'S HEART

Although there are a large number of horizontal studies comparing trained and nontrained persons, there are surprisingly few longitudinal studies to answer the questions concerning the development and regression of the athlete's heart. The following questions, therefore, cannot be definitively answered at this time.

1. Is there a genetic predisposition for the development of athlete's heart and, if so, how can this be recognized? Given the appropriate training, can every heart reach a volume of 1,700 ml, or is this reserved for the children with unexpectedly large and obviously healthy hearts, who later develop into olympic winners in the endurance sports? This has been suggested repeatedly, although we may have to look for other indicators in trying to predict the ability to become a major endurance athlete.

2. At what age does physiologic hypertrophy develop? There is no question that this can occur in the postpubertal period of growth. There is a great debate in the literature whether the athlete's heart can start to develop before puberty, whether the cardiac size continues to in-

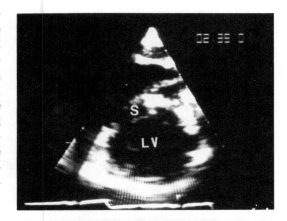

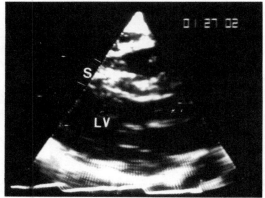

FIG 3–10.
Example of a thickened septum in a totally symptom-free swimmer. Shown by two-dimensional echocardiography from our data obtained by Satomi (in preparation). Left ventricular cross section *(top)* and two-chamber view *(bottom)*. *LV,* left ventricle; *S,* septum.

crease if the athlete continues to train beyond the 20th year, and whether an athlete's heart can develop in a person who does not begin to train until after the 40th year of life.

3. Is there, or is there not, a complete regression of the athlete's heart after the training stops? If there is no total regression, is this due to an irreversible growth of the framework of the heart, or do these hearts remain large because of the sustained, although minimal, physical activity of the ex-athlete, who still maintains an increased potential for physical activity?

The answer to these questions is based largely on opinion and not on fact. The reason for this is evident. Concerning the development of the athlete's heart, it is based on the uncertainty as to which one of the very many youngsters entering a particular area of athletics is going to succeed as a champion in that field. It is obviously not possible to examine all the youthful athletes and without this, a definitive answer to this question is most unlikely. As far as the regression of the athlete's heart is concerned, it seems extremely unlikely that a highly-trained athlete should completely give up all physical activity and thus make it possible to observe regression, without any outside influence.

The three questions raised above can be answered in the following fashion.

1. There is general agreement in the literature that the primary determinant of the maximal oxygen uptake is heredity. However, to what percentage genetics play a role in this process is widely debated. While Weber (1976) and Ekblom (1968) believe that hereditary factors are responsible for 50% of the maximal oxygen uptake, Astrand (1969) believes that only 20% of the maximal oxygen uptake can be modified by training and Klissouras (1971) believes that this portion is less than 10%. Unfortunately, there is no study to show the role of hereditary factors as a subdivision of the metabolic and cardiocirculatory components. The question of whether the maximal oxygen uptake is due to the number of red muscle fibers, which are probably genetically determined, or directly to some genetic cardiocirculatory factors cannot yet be answered. Even though we accept the thesis that every heart cannot develop into an extreme athlete's heart, we still don't know whether this is due to an inherent limitation of the growth potential or to a genetically controlled limitation in the maximal muscular oxygen utilization that then secondarily limits the cardiac growth potential.

2. One glance at the literature shows that Reindell (1960) had found that the hypertrophy of the heart depended to a large extent on the intensity of the training, even in adults. In contrast, Czermak (1970) believes that a physiologic cardiac hypertrophy can occur only in the young. This belief was endorsed by Grimby (1966), who did not find larger hearts in athletes who continued their training into the fifth and sixth decade, when compared to younger athletes. He concluded that in adults the heart did not enlarge further.

Others have believed for a long time that the circulation could not be trained prior to puberty. This view was based on the fact that in training experiments that compared children with control groups, the circulatory functional capacity could not be increased. On the basis of his own studies, Schmucker (1973) developed the hypothesis that this was due to a lack of sufficient hormones. It is known that for a hypertrophy of skeletal muscle to occur, an appropriate testosterone level was necessary. The inability to train the heart prior to puberty can be considered as an analogous situation. The animal experiments of Beznak (1960) and Goldberg (1969) support the thesis that the ability to train the heart depends on the presence of an adequate testosterone level. Wasmund (1972) and other groups in Germany, and Bar-or (1972) in Israel found also that the heart could not be trained in children. This is in contrast to the findings of investigators in the German Democratic Republic and Eastern Europe in general, who did find that the heart could be trained in children (Oelschlägel, 1976; Leupold, 1969). Nevertheless, the inability to train the heart in children prior to puberty is still considered to be a dogma in training theory.

On the other hand, this view can no longer be reconciled with the current developments in high-performance athletics. We now find an increasing shift of the age of high performance toward earlier childhood and in swimming, even including the endurance trials. When children prior to puberty can engage in daily swimming sessions of 4–5 hours, this can no longer be attributed to a drive toward a better swimming technique. Our own investigations, shown in Figure 3–11, reveal that an increased maximal oxygen uptake occurs in children of 8 to 10 years of age, accompanied by a corresponding increase in the volume of the heart and an increase in the internal diameter of the heart and in the thickness of the heart wall, as proved by echocardiography. These obviously are clear indications of the development of the athlete's heart.

The fact that in other investigations the effect of training could not be demonstrated is probably due to the fact that the nontrained control group was also engaging in considerable physical activity. It seems likely that the above-cited studies relied too heavily on comparisons with conditions found in the adults. Since the average citizen is at a "zero-training" status, even very minor training activity can lead to improvements of performance. Children, on the other hand, are continuously in motion, and thus there is never, or hardly ever, a totally nontrained child. It is also true in training theory that the lower the starting level, the easier it is to achieve some training results. The effects of training, therefore, can be seen in children only after a comparatively much higher training effort. This actually is not due to the fact that children are more difficult to train, but to the fact that there is no truly "nontrained" control group.

On the other hand, it could be argued that considering the greater plasticity of the young heart, early training may well lead to athlete's hearts, even larger than those seen to date. Our longitudinal studies, extending now over a period of 10 years, have shown no evidence to support such a theory in the children we had studied. In spite of the earlier start of the training period, the swimmers did not demonstrate hearts any larger than usually found in athletes in this sport. These findings can be considered as further support for the concept of the critical heart size. The longitudinal study in children further shows that there was no evidence to suggest that the early start of high-performance training had any bearing on the development of cardiac damage. It can therefore be stated from a cardiology point of view that endurance

---

FIG 3–11.

Data from our cross-sectional and longitudinal studies in prepubertal children (from our study group, by Gerhardus, 1980). The *cross-hatched* columns represent groups of 8-, 9-, and 10-year-old children who were engaged in competitive swimming. The values obtained at the control time *(first column)* were compared with data obtained 1 year later *(second column)*. Every age group contained six boys and six girls who are grouped together since there were no statistically significant sex-related differences between the groups. This group was compared to a comparable group of school children *(clear columns)*. As the data indicate, there is an evident absolute and relative increase in oxygen uptake even in prepubertal children **(a).** The increase in oxygen uptake is accompanied by a corresponding absolute and relative increase in cardiac volume **(b).** The echocardiographic findings indicate that this increase in cardiac volume is not a simple dilatation, but a true adaptation process. Not only the left ventricular internal diameter is increased $(LVID_d)$ but the thickness of the left ventricular wall is thickened as well $(LVWD_d)$. In cross-sectional studies in prepubertal children in the 8–10 year age groups, there is clear evidence of a development of the athlete's heart when compared to a nontrained group. The longitudinal studies show that the performance capacity and the cardiac size are increasing much more than could be expected by age alone.

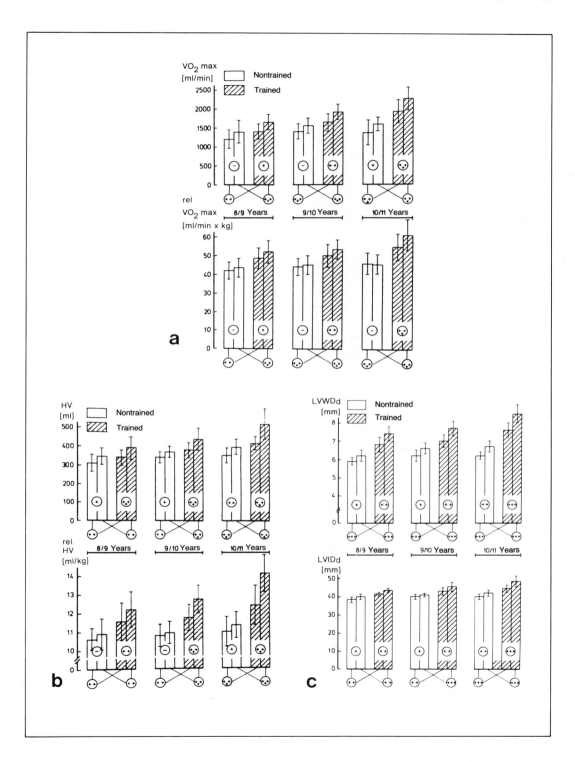

stress, even starting at an early age, does not cause cardiac damage. The question of whether it is proper to impose such a burden on children at an early age, cannot be answered from studies of this kind. This is a question that must be decided on educational grounds.

The question concerning the feasability of cardiopulmonary training in children, which was discussed to date mostly on the grounds of its endurance-performance athletic merits, was recently given a new dimension. Is it reasonable for children to engage in endurance training in the framework of societal or school athletics, in order to prevent the cardiovascular problems of older age? This argument was countered in the past with reference to the above studies, which claimed that the hearts of children could not be trained anyway. While our studies show that the effect of training can indeed be demonstrated in the cardiocirculatory system of children, it is questionable if the already high, normal activity of children could be much enhanced by having them run once or twice a week in school.

There are also other considerations that may argue against involving children in endurance training (e.g., long distance running, perhaps even up to the marathon distance). Children are not threatened by ischemic heart disease and endurance training is contrary to the normal, play-oriented mentality of childhood. Furthermore, involving children in training of many hours' duration may take them away from other athletic activities such as gymnastics or games that would be more suitable from educational and health points of view. Today children are particularly prone to postural defects that in later life may lead to spinal column deformities. From an athletic-educational point of view, children should be offered a variety of activity options, so they can use their highly coordinated learning ability and pick the

form of athletics that is particularly suited for themselves.

The same argument, however, can also be used to begin the endurance training already in school. The child should learn that endurance training is an important part of physical conditioning. It makes no sense for a 40-year-old, who has been abusing tobacco for 20 years and who has never engaged in physical activity, to start running at that age after the first symptoms of cardiac pathology have appeared. Children should be made to realize that endurance training is just as important as all the other aspects of physical hygiene. The introduction of the endurance training in school should be primarily for informational purposes and not, as it is unfortunately done too often, for the purposes of achieving a high performance. In children who are not physically or emotionally prepared for this, the effect may be a strongly negative motivation.

3. The *regression of the athlete's heart* was studied in 19 older ex-athletes by Holmgren (1959) and in 92 such persons by Roskamm (1964). Both investigators reached the same conclusion. The hearts of these former athletes were still larger than those of untrained controls, even when the athletes have discontinued all physical activity. On the other hand, the functional capacity of the experimental subjects was also greater. It may come as a surprise to those who believe that athletics has only beneficial effects that the ECGs of these former athletes showed a statistically nonsignificant, but frequent, increase in abnormalities when compared to the control group.

As already discussed, the question must be raised as to whether we are dealing with a permanent, irreversible enlargement of the supporting structures of the heart or with an expression of a sustained increase in functional capacity. The fact that some of these athletes engaged in no physical activity at all suggests that the thesis that even normal physical activity is sufficient to maintain the increased performance ability is correct. It could also be true that in this group of athletes, we were dealing with a select group that is capable of a high performance even without training.

The problems introduced by factors in selection can be seen particularly well in Holmgren's data. His studies showed that eight of the 19 former athletes examined by him, i.e., a high percentage, had pathologic findings on both the resting and stress ECGs. In comparison to a younger group of athletes, the size of the heart was practically the same, i.e., significantly larger than in the untrained. The functional capacity was elevated for their age, but was not increased to the same extent as the size of their heart volume. The conclusion can be drawn that ECG changes are frequently seen later in life in athletes and that the size of the fully developed athlete's heart does not regress. These two conclusions can be taken together to formulate the theory that the fully developed athlete's heart is prone to suffer cardiac illness later in life. To put this interpretation in its proper perspective, we must appreciate the additional information, namely that the 19 former athletes who were examined were those who volunteered from a group of 44 athletes invited to do so. It seems likely, therefore, that the athletes who took advantage of the opportunity for such a diagnostic evaluation were those who suffered from cardiac symptoms. If this is true, then the above findings are the result of a sampling error.

The question whether the athlete's heart has the ability to regress is usually answered from the general prejudicial point of view that was discussed at length above. In discussions with athletes and sports physicians the concept fre-

quently emerges that the owner of an athlete's heart has to continue to run to avoid a myocardial infarct. This concept is totally wrong. Even though it is very difficult to answer the question of whether the athlete's heart can regress completely or not, since very few athletes stop all physical activity completely at the end of their athletic career, there is no fundamental difference in the regression of the trained heart muscle and the regression of skeletal muscle. This can be supported by the observation made by our group that the largest athlete's heart ever measured (1,700 ml) regressed to a normal volume of 980 ml in 10 years, after its owner completed his athletic career.

During this regression phase cardiac symptoms, even premature beats at rest, are frequent and cause considerable anxiety in the endurance athletes, who generally are very conscious of their physical well-being. These complaints, which in no way represent any organic danger, should be classified as the *athletic withdrawal syndrome* and should form the basis for the recommendation that the intense training activity in the athlete should be tapered slowly over a period of time. Such a recommendation is particularly suitable to the athletes who engage in athletics for the pleasure of the exercise, even when they are no longer engaged in endurance training for competitive purposes. If the athlete has to stop all physical activity abruptly, he can be reassured that there is no cardiac danger in so doing. Even the athlete who must spend 6 months flat on his back following a complicated fracture of the leg does not have an infarct on this basis.

THE FUNCTION OF THE ATHLETE'S HEART

Function of the Athlete's Heart at Rest

Henschen was not only the first one to describe the athlete's heart, but he was also the first one to discuss the particular aspects of its function. According to his observations, the athletes had a high pulse amplitude that suggested that they had large and strong hearts. This observation leads to the hemodynamic conclusion that the athlete's heart has a large stroke volume. This is in marked contrast to the presumed function of the athlete's heart, which is presented below.

It is surprising, however, that the studies of Henschen make no reference to the chief characteristic of the athlete's heart, i.e., *training bradycardia*. This can be explained by the fact that all his investigations took place under prestart conditions, i.e., before the start of a race or contest. Training bradycardia can be very pronounced. Rates of less than 30 beats per minute have been described. The lowest rate observed by us was 26 beats per minute, found during sleep by Holter monitoring (Fig 3–12). The lowest rate recorded in the literature, obtained under similar conditions, was 21 beats per minute (Zeppilli, 1981).

It is surprising that these very low rates are generally based on a regular sinus rhythm. Israel (1975) has pointed out that escape rhythms are relatively rare. The degree of bradycardia is but a very poor measure of the level of training. The resting rate is influenced to a great extent by psychic factors. Very low rates can also be found occasionally in nontrained people who have a high vagal tone. It is not totally surprising that of nine German athletic teams, the gymnasts have the lowest rate, even though these athletes have a comparatively low cardiovascular functional capacity (Roskamm, 1964).

Although the training bradycardia is a very striking phenomenon, it has not been adequately elucidated to date. In order to explain it, two apparently contradictory models can be used that may, however, interact in a supplementary fashion. Training bradycardia may be the result of a very large stroke volume, as suggested by Frick (1967), or it is possible that the heart rate is controlled primarily by peripheral mechanisms. This was proposed by Stegemann and his coworkers (1974). From this latter point of view, the large stroke volume should be considered as the consequence and not the cause of the low heart rate.

To integrate these two apparently contradictory points of view, we may have to start out from the concept of a regulatory circle. The increased stroke volume probably reduces the nervous impulses to the heart, in the form of a "negative feedback" and lowers the heart rate. In this way, the two components of the cardiac output, i.e., the heart rate and the stroke volume, affect each other. The above-described relative independence of the training bradycardia from the cardiac performance, and the fact that in mass athletic activity, bradycardia can be observed without cardiac enlargement, seem to contradict the thesis of Frick, according to which the athlete's heart can afford a low heart rate because it has a large stroke volume. These observations suggest that the regulation of the heart

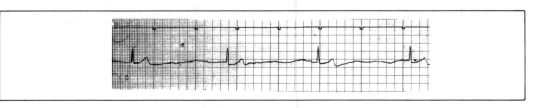

FIG 3–12.

Example of extreme bradycardia in an athlete's heart, obtained during sleep by Holter monitoring. This strip shows a heart rate of 26 beats per minute in a water polo player.

rate must be under the control of autonomic nervous influences. On the other hand, the same observations do not necessarily exclude the possibility that the above-described feedback mechanism permits the increased stroke volume to influence the heart rate. In regard to the autonomic nervous control of the heart rate, we must distinguish between resting and stress conditions. The decreased heart rate in the trained individual under stress conditions can be attributed, without any difficulty, to a decrease in sympathetic stimulation. In contrast, the decrease in the heart rate under resting conditions is usually regarded as the result of an increased vagal tone. In this regard, it is usually forgotten that such a massive bradycardia (30 beats per minute) can hardly be due to a general increase in *vagal tone*. If this were the case, an increased vagal tone should be manifest in the noncardiac areas, e.g., a dilated pupil, increased salivation, etc.

To understand the *etiology of the training bradycardia*, some animal experiments, particularly those of Tipton (1965), may be helpful. They indicate that for the onset of a bradycardia, myocardial changes must be present. It can be shown that in trained rats there is a decrease in heart rate even if the heart is isolated from the autonomic nervous system. According to these findings, the heart rate is diminished not through an increase in the vagal tone, but by an increased sensitivity of the heart to vagal stimulation. The atrial muscle of the trained rat can be shown to contain an increased concentration of unbound acetylcholine. It seems likely that in the trained individual a combination of an increased vagal tone and an increased sensitivity of the heart to vagal stimulation may be additive in the etiology of training bradycardia.

As far as the *clinical evaluation of training bradycardia* is concerned, it can be established that in the endurance-trained athlete, an increased stroke volume can compensate without any difficulty for the decreased heart rate. Even high-performance athletes have no problems attributable to the extreme bradycardia. The training bradycardia must therefore be considered as a physiologic process. This still begs the question, however, in clinical medicine, as to whether the responsiveness of the heart to vagal tone may not be an additional pathogenetic factor leading to a situation where a patient literally "runs himself" into the need for an artificial pacemaker. Even though there is no evidence that training bradycardia can progress to the point where it produces a syncopal attack, there have been cases in which there was a high index of suspicion that the vagal effects due to training may have contributed to organic or functional cardiac disturbances and therefore had to be considered to be pathogenetic.

This suspicion is demonstrated by a single observation. We studied a 46-year-old patient who had been running long distances for 5 years, who had five to six training sessions per week, and who ran the marathon distance in 3 hours. It was known that he had a slow heart rate since childhood and that this rate was further diminished to a low of 30 beats per minute during training. The patient came to our attention when he complained of premature beats and dyspnea mostly during rest. In one of these episodes, when he had severe dyspnea at night, his pulse rate was 30 beats per minute. He could barely walk, but under these conditions the symptoms were markedly decreased. He then stopped running completely and his pulse rate rose to 54 beats per minute. An intensive cardiac diagnostic work-up, including a *bundle of His ECG*, failed to reveal any cardiac pathology. The tentative diagnosis was one of an isolated sinus node damage, superimposed by exercise-induced vagal sensitivity, which resulted in a critical bradycardia. This patient had diptheria as a child. The patient was advised to discontinue long-distance running.

On the basis of this case it must be assumed that in the presence of a moderately severe but distinct sick sinus syndrome, clinically significant bradycardia can be triggered by an increased vagal tone, superimposed by exercise. This assumption is made even more likely when we realize that there are clinical observations (Treese, 1982) that strongly suggest that the sick sinus syndrome must be regarded as a functional disturbance of the autonomic nervous system. Such observations are relatively common in sports cardiology research institutions. The assumption that increased vagal effects, added to an underlying conduction defect, may lead to a third degree heart block and the need for an implanted pacemaker is substantiated by a case report by Franz (1979). In a 59-year-old patient who had always engaged in athletics (tennis, long-distance running, and swimming), the first diagnostic work-up revealed a sinus bradycardia, a first degree atrioventricular (AV) block, e.g., a PQ interval of 0.28 seconds and a conduction time shortened by exercise to 0.16 seconds. Eighteen months later he showed a PQ interval of 0.34 and a Wenckebach periodicity. Another 18 months later he reported Stokes-Adams attacks, had a third degree heart block, and required the insertion of a pacemaker.

Such observations can usually be made only in older patients and only very rarely in young ones. It is precisely in the older patient who engages in endurance sports and who has a bradycardia that the clinical question arises as to whether this is a functional disturbance of the sinus node or a simple training effect. The stress ECG is helpful in this situation. If it is a functional disturbance of the sinus node, there will be only an inadequate rise in pulse rate, even under maximal stress. The age-dependent maximal rate of 200, minus the age in years, cannot be attained. Instead we see compensatory premature beats even under moderate stress, and sinus arrhythmias that are ordinarily not seen under stress (Fig 3–13).

If the question is raised as to whether an insufficient rise in heart rate in the older man under stress is due to a functional sinus node injury or to insufficient strength to handle the stress, a determination of the lactate level is helpful. If the inadequate rise in heart rate is due to cardiac causes, a high lactate level will be found even at relatively low pulse rates, indicating a significantly low level of metabolic activity.

If there is evidence that the effect of training on the pulse rate may contribute to pathogenesis, one must draw the appropriate conclusions and advise the affected athlete to refrain from any further endurance exercise. They should be guided toward less demanding game-athletics like tennis, gymnastics, etc., although this may be difficult to accomplish in a dedicated long-distance runner.

While there is no question about the effects of training on cardiac rate, and even though the interpretation of training bradycardia may present problems, there was considerable debate in the past about the second component of the cardiac output, i.e., *stroke volume*. This debate is of interest not only for the athlete's heart but also for the fundamental regulation of cardiac work, since, based on findings made in the athlete's heart, the validity of the Starling mechanism was questioned even for the healthy heart.

As discussed in regard to the regulation of cardiac work under stress conditions, the Starling mechanism does not play a major role in the adaptation of the cardiocirculatory system to stress. The importance of the Starling mechanism as the all-important single factor in increas-

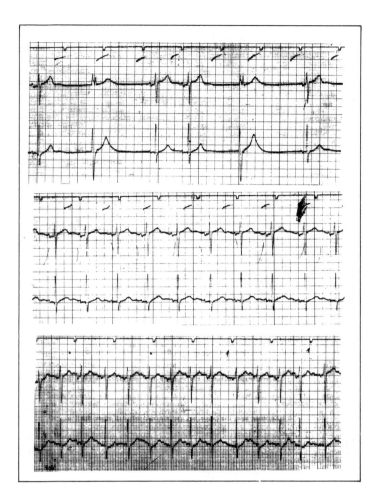

FIG 3–13.
This electrocardiogram (ECG) is an example of the problems encountered in the interpretation of "training-dependent" ECG changes, particularly in the elderly person. It was taken in a 55-year-old long-distance runner. The *two top strips* were taken at rest and clearly show a sinus bradycardia and extra beats (2 and 4 cardiac action). Such changes can appear in the young athlete as a consequence of training. In the older athlete, the question must be asked whether this represents the effects of conditioning or whether this is a sign of sinus node disease. The stress ECG is helpful in this dilemma. After moderate load we see an increase in rate *(middle).* Under heavy load *(bottom)* the rate does not rise above 120 beats per minute and a sinus arrhythmia appears that does not occur normally on the stress ECG. These changes are strongly suggestive of sinus node disease.

ing the stroke volume is further weakened by the findings in the athlete's heart that show that the increase in stroke volume was due to an increase in heart size and not to increased filling. This mechanism for the increase in stroke volume was described by Reindell with the term *regulatory cardiac enlargement.* Reindell emphasizes that such adaptation occurs not only under physiologic high stress conditions, but also under conditions of increased volume work as seen under pathologic conditions such as septal defects and valvular lesions.

In the German literature of the 1950s this led to a surprising conclusion concerning the athlete's heart. It almost totally eliminated the Starling mechanism from any consideration. In spite of the view of Henschen, who attributed to the athlete's heart a high stroke volume, it was assumed that the resting stroke volume of the athlete's heart was not enlarged and, indeed, that it was reduced. This view was based on noninvasive diagnostic techniques, e.g., sphygmography, ballistocardiography, and others (Christensen, 1937; Jokl, 1959; Reindell, 1960; Israel, 1968). Even though these results could not be duplicated by later, invasive techniques and have therefore only a historic significance, they will be discussed briefly since they still influence some current thinking concerning the function of the athlete's heart, but more importantly, because they illustrate one of the fundamental problems in sports cardiology: the question of research methodology.

The advances in general cardiology have been made for some time now, through the use of invasive techniques such as catheterizations that are clearly inappropriate in healthy young athletes. In athletes the studies were performed with the less reliable noninvasive techniques. Excessive reliance on data so obtained inevitably led to erroneous conclusions. Fortunately for sports medicine this situation has recently undergone significant changes. Cardiology today has access to highly reliable, very sensitive, noninvasive research methodologies, such as echocardiography, nuclear medicine studies, computer-assisted tomography, etc., all of which are of great benefit to research and should be even more welcome to sports medicine than to general cardiology. We have to be cautious, however, not to place undue reliance on these new techniques and repeat the mistakes made in sports medicine in the past, but on a more sophisticated level.

The findings obtained with these techniques, i.e., the smaller stroke volume in the enlarged athlete's heart as compared to the smaller, nontrained

heart, cannot be explained on the basis of the Starling mechanism, particularly if we take into account the data from stress research. Research data obtained through invasive techniques (Bevegard, 1963; Musshoff, 1959) indicate that the athlete's heart has a greater stroke volume under stress than the nontrained heart, even though its filling pressure and heart size do not change as compared to the resting state. Bevegard did find a slight increase in end-diastolic pressure in athletes that he attributed to a decreased compliance of the hypertrophied athlete's heart. This finding could not be substantiated by the research group in Freiburg (see Kindermann, 1974). It was deduced from these observations that the Starling mechanism was valid only in animal experiments or in the sick heart. So-called "New Laws of the Heart" were postulated. Wezler (1969) used these findings in athlete's heart to evolve his hypothesis concerning the active diastolic tone of cardiac muscle. He assumed that in diastole the myocardium could adapt through autoregulation in a plastic fashion to different levels of filling.

As can be seen in Reindell's description (1960), the following hemodynamic model was assumed: the athlete's heart functions at rest not only at an unusually low rate, but also at a very low stroke volume. This results in a particularly small cardiac output. This decrease in cardiac output was allegedly made possible by an increased metabolic capacity of the trained skeletal muscle, i.e., a high arteriovenous oxygen gradient. This was taken to be a sign of the particularly notable effectiveness of the trained circulation. A low stroke volume combined with a large left ventricle must go hand in hand with a high end-systolic blood volume (resting blood), and a low ejection fraction. According to the Starling mechanism, increased end-systolic volume must lead to a large stroke volume in the healthy heart. According to this view, and on this basis, the end-systolic ventricular volume lost its importance as a regulatory factor and was considered only as a reserve volume that was necessary in the transition phase between the beginning of increased work and the appearance of an increased venous return.

The results of our investigations (Rost, 1979; Schneider, 1970), using the dye-dilution technique, could not substantiate the presence of a low stroke volume as a function of the increased heart size (Fig 3–14). On the other hand, the *cardiac output* at rest was slightly less in the trained individual, as compared to the nontrained one. The nontrained young men had a cardiac output of 3.881 L/min/m^2 of body surface (cardiac index). The same value in athletes having bradycardia of less than 60 beats per minute averaged 3.231 L/min.

Musshoff reported similar findings. In his studies the Nylin index was 9.17 in the nontrained persons and 10.33 in the athletes. This means that in the athlete the resting volume was less than in the nontrained person, when related to heart size. On this basis it can be stated that, while the resting stroke volume is absolutely greater in the athlete than in the nontrained person, this is insufficient to compensate for the bradycardia. The slightly diminished cardiac output in the trained person can be attributed to the decreased venous return. This latter is probably due to venous distentions, presumably due to an increase in the vagal tone. Using invasive techniques, other investigators (Astrand, 1964; Bevegard, 1963; Grimby, 1966; Kindermann, 1974) have also found an increased stroke volume in the athletes. These studies were open to some questions such as whether arterial puncture and cardiac catheterization were compatible with the "resting state." On this basis, echocardiography, which provided a new dimension to the noninvasive evaluation of cardiac function, has assumed particular importance.

If the older view concerning the function of the athlete's heart is correct, one would expect that the athlete's heart at rest demonstrated only very slight wall motion, as compared to the motion seen under stress conditions. Such findings were alleged with radiologic-kymographic studies and were used as proof for the thesis. Unfortunately, they could not be substantiated by echocardiographic means. The examples shown in Figure 3–15,A prove unmistakeably that at rest, the wall of the athlete's heart moves significantly and that this movement is essentially of the same order of magnitude as under stress conditions. Therefore, since the athlete's heart has an increased ventricular diameter, its stroke volume must be well above the average, even at rest.

In view of these qualitative findings by *echocardiography*, the question remains whether this technique can be used for quantitative evaluation of the stroke volume. There are a number of different formulas that can be used by investigators and that are of particular significance in sports medicine by virtue of the importance of using noninvasive techniques. Among the many formulas for the calculation of stroke volume by echocardiography, the "elipsoid model" of Feigenbaum (1972) is the most widely applicable. According to this model, the stroke volume is calculated to be the difference between the cube of the systolic and diastolic diameter of the left ventricle. The problem of determining stroke volume echocardiographically by the M-mode technique lies in the fact that this technique attempts to draw conclusions about a complicated three-dimensional structure like the left ventricle on the basis of a unidimensional measurement like the diameter of the left ventricle. Such a process assumes a number of conditions that cannot all be met, as was stated forcefully in a critique by Linhart (1975).

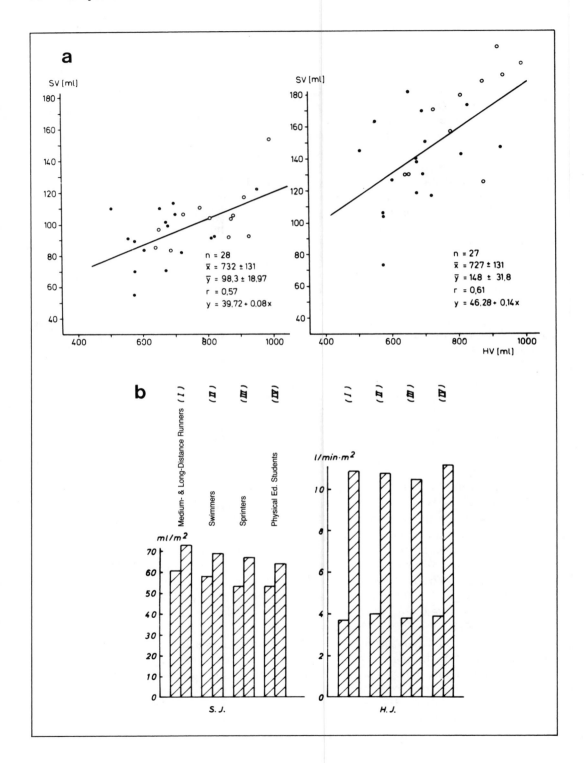

His criticisms are summarized in a well-known publication that has the provocative title: "Left ventricular volume measurements by echocardiography: fact or fiction?" His answer to this question was, "Fiction!"

It is thus a philosophical question whether or not one accepts echocardiography as a tool in the measurement of stroke volume. Those authors who answer this question in the affirmative rest their case on the nice correlations between echocardiographic findings and findings by other techniques as demonstrated by Feigenbaum. On the other hand, a quote from Feigenbaum should dampen any excessive enthusiasm. He entitled his first publication on the use of echocardiography for the determination of stroke volume: "Use of ultrasound, to *measure* left ventricular stroke volume."

In a newer review on the same subject (1975) he wrote: "The fact is, that *echocardiography does not measure left ventricular volumes* . . . if one assumes that the left ventricle is contracting symmetrically and that it is roughly an ellipsoid with a uniform shape, then there is a statistical correlation between the dimensions and the corresponding volumes." In spite of such moderation voiced by the echocardiographers, this technique is used relatively uncritically in sports medicine. Measurements of

stroke volume are reported in a number of publications. The same is true for the determination of left ventricular muscle mass, which is based on the same model. According to our own results, the "cube" formula gives exaggerated stroke volume values, since the athlete's heart does not have a ratio of 2:1 between the long axis and the short axis of the left ventricle and thus differs from the standard ellipsoid model. In the athlete's heart, the shape of the left ventricle is more circular as it is in all enlarged hearts, and thus, the given ratio is smaller. Howald (1977) used the Teichholz equation, which contains a correction factor for such deviations. On the other hand Simon (1981) found reasonable values for stroke volume in athletes, using the "cube" formula. According to him, this was due to a better selection of the moment for determining the end-diastolic diameter.

If one reviews the discussions concerning the resting stroke volume in the trained athlete, one can decide that it is increased, contrary to earlier opinions. Considering its size, the athlete's heart functions according to the same laws as the normal heart. This means that the Starling mechanism is operative, even though it is affected by extracardiac factors. The debate was caused by methodological problems, i.e., an underestimation of the stroke volume by noninvasive

---

FIG 3–14.
This figure demonstrates the effects of physical conditioning on the relationship between cardiac size and volume work. The data are derived from our own studies and the cardiac output and stroke volume were determined by the dye-dilution technique. **a,** the relationship between cardiac size, measured as cardiac volume and stroke volume *(SV)*. The *solid dots* represent data from nontrained persons; the *circles* are data obtained from trained athletes. On the *left* the resting stroke volume is plotted against cardiac size, on the *right* the plot is between exercise stroke volume and cardiac size. The relationship between stroke volume and cardiac size is apparent and becomes even more obvious under exercise. **b,** the

stroke index (stroke volume/surface area in m²) on the *left,* and the cardiac index (cardiac output/surface area in m²) on the *right*. The first column shows the resting values and the second column shows the values during ergometer exercise in the supine position at 210-watt load. Observe that the resting and exercise stroke volume is clearly related to the level of endurance training. The highest values are shown by the middle- and long-distance runners; the lowest values are shown by the relatively untrained students. In contrast, there is no relationship between cardiac output at rest or during exercise and the level of training.

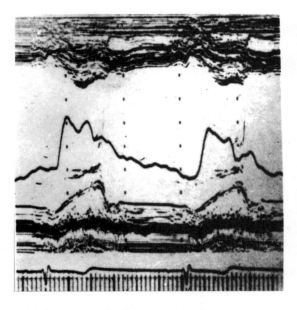
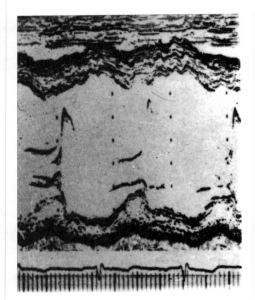
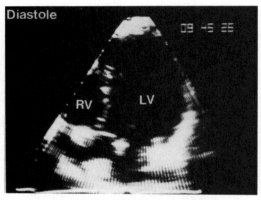
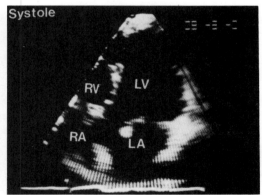
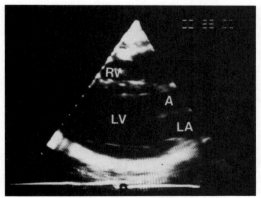
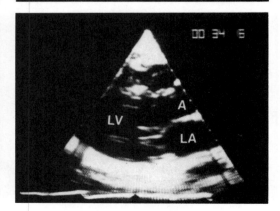

techniques. This should serve as a warning not to repeat old mistakes with new techniques, such as echocardiography. The use of echocardiography in the determination of the stroke volume is of particular interest in regard to the athlete's heart. The issue is not yet resolved, and it is possible that the introduction of the two-dimensional echocardiography will give a new impetus to this matter. The currrently available findings obtained by *two-dimensional echocardiographic determinations of stroke volume* at rest and under stress conditions still indicate methodologic problems (Fig 3–15,B). The size of the stroke volume is underestimated due to the fact that the long axis of the left ventricle is measured at an angle, and hence is also underestimated.

Function of the Athlete's Heart Under Physical Exercise

The first statement about the function of the athlete's heart under exercise conditions was made by Krogh in 1913. Krogh believed that a trained heart could increase its ejection volume to 20 L/min under stress. In fact, this is only about 50% of the real, maximal cardiac output that can be obtained by the optimally trained, endurance athlete, through, as we now know, improved investigational methods. Using the dye-dilution technique, Ekblom (1968) described the highest recorded *cardiac output* at 42.3 L/min. This finding agrees well with some older findings by Christensen (1931, 1937) who found a rise in the cardiac

output to 37 L/min, using the "foreign gas" technique. Although Krogh grossly underestimated the relative performance potential of the athlete's heart in absolute numbers, he recognized the relative increase accurately, since he started from a resting output of only 3 L/min.

This twofold increase in cardiac output, as compared to the values in the untrained heart, is accomplished by an increase in the *stroke volume*. A frequently encountered error starts from the assumption that the trained heart is capable of higher rates than the nontrained one. In fact, the *maximal rate* is determined by biologic factors, such as age, and is totally independent from the level of physical conditioning. The trained heart not only does not achieve a higher rate, but since the maximal rate is, to some extent, a function of the heart size, it is usually somewhat less in the endurance trained athlete than in the nontrained person (Ekblom, 1968).

This means that the athlete's heart must reach stroke volumes in the 200 ml range under conditions of stress. In fact, the largest stroke volume recorded by Ekblom was 205 ml. Thus, a large stroke volume is the characteristic hemodynamic feature of the trained circulation. The same cardiac work can be accomplished with a lower cardiac rate, since, given the same intensity of stress, the cardiac output is the same in the trained and nontrained person. Since for any given level of exercise the efficiency, i.e., oxygen uptake, is independent of the level of training, the oxygen utilization, i.e., the

FIG 3–15.
Two echocardiograms at rest and during exercise are shown. **Top,** M-mode echocardiogram in a very good bicycle racer. The *left side* of the echo shows the resting curve and also the carotid wave form. The *right side* was obtained during physical exercise on the bicycle ergometer in the supine position. The tracing shows clearly that the diameter of the left ventricle is only minimally reduced during exercise. The

amount of wall motion is almost identical during rest and under exercise. **Bottom,** two-dimensional representation of the motion of the heart in an athlete. *Left,* diastole; *right,* systole, *above* in the so-called four-chamber view. **Below,** the two-chamber view. *RV,* right ventricle; *LV,* left ventricle; *RA,* right atrium; *LA,* left atrium; *A,* aorta.

arterio-venous oxygen gradient, should be essentially the same in the trained and nontrained person under identical conditions of stress.

The above hemodynamic model can be substantiated by studies done with invasive diagnostic techniques (Astrand, 1964; Ekblom, 1968). Our own studies led to the same results (Rost, 1979; Schneider, 1970). Even on this point, however, the frequently encountered general views concerning the functioning of the trained circulation differ from the data found in the literature. It is generally assumed that because of better metabolic function and better enzymatic adaptation of the musculature, the trained circulation can perform better by utilizing more of the arterial oxygen content. In complete contrast to this view, a number of authors have found, on the basis of invasive techniques, that under load conditions the trained heart demonstrated a hyperkinetic behavior. In other words, they found an increased cardiac output and a decreased arteriovenous oxygen gradient, under identical conditions of stress (Bevegard, 1963; Grimby, 1966; Kindermann, 1974). There are very few studies that support the view of an increased oxygen utilization (Hanson, 1965). The latter studies were done with the subject on the treadmill, so that it is possible that a performer with a better running technique could show a decreased oxygen requirement and, therefore, a lower cardiac output.

The findings reported on the basis of noninvasive techniques will not be considered in this discussion, since under these conditions the very rapid circulatory flow rate could lead to even greater error than under conditions of rest. In the older literature and even in the more recent literature, particularly American literature, studies that usually employ the indirect Fick technique showed a decrease in cardiac output under identical stress conditions (Andrew, 1966; Krogh,

1913; Lindhard, 1915). The opposite can also be found in the literature (Bock, 1928). In spite of such findings, and considering only the data which were obtained by invasive techniques, it can be stated that under submaximal stress conditions the trained heart does not decrease the volume work of the heart by increasing oxygen utilization. This opinion is contrary to the findings made in a number of studies on peripheral perfusion. *Plethysmographic studies* showed that after training, the peripheral perfusion decreased by 30% to 50% (Schroeder, 1972).

As a criticism of these studies it must be stated that plethysmographic studies can be performed only after the exercise is over. It is therefore interesting to point out that the first investigator who found a decrease in muscle perfusion in athletes after exercise with a plethysmographic technique reached a contrary conclusion (Elsner, 1962). In his view, the decreased perfusion after exercise is an indication of increased perfusion during exercise.

Studies performed with the xenon technique, which can be used even during exercise, were used to justify the extrapolation of postexercise findings by plethysmography to the state of affairs during the period of exercise (Clausen, 1970). On the other hand, the range of scatter is so great with the xenon technique, that its use can really not be justified. A decrease of the perfusion, as a consequence of training, seems very unlikely on the basis of oxygen utilization studies as well. Doll (1968) found no difference in the oxygen saturation of femoral venous blood between athletes and nonathletes.

While *cross sectional studies* consistently show no difference in cardiac output between trained and nontrained persons after conditions of similar stress, longitudinal studies gave entirely different results. A number of authors found a decrease in cardiac output under similar stress conditions, even after a relatively short training period (Andrew, 1966; Clausen, 1969; Ekblom, 1968; Saltin, 1968). Even though these findings could not be substantiated by other authors (Freedman, 1955; Frick, 1963; Hartley, 1968, 1969), including our own studies published by Dreisbach (1976), it must be emphasized that there may well be differences between the effects of a relatively short training period and the effects of a high-performance training period lasting several years.

The findings of Ekblom permit us to draw the following conclusions: Under similar stress intensities, at the beginning of training there will be a decrease in cardiac output and a simultaneous increase in the arteriovenous oxygen gradient. This means that initially there will be an increased metabolic capacity of the skeletal muscles and an increased utilization of the capillary network, at least as long as there is no dimensional adaptation of the cardiac size. In the later stages of training, after at least 1 year of intensive conditioning, there is a *dimensional adaptation*, and the cardiac size increases. At this point, an increased stroke volume produces a cardiac output which once again makes the cardiac output similar between the trained and the nontrained performer.

Since these results are so contradictory and since they are of relatively minor significance for the athlete's heart, they will not be discussed further at this point. Their significance in the context of cardiac rehabilitation training is discussed in the section on "Physical Conditioning in the Prevention of Cardiac Disease."

The discussion concerning the effects of training prior to the development of the athlete's heart shows that one of the characteristic features of the athlete's heart, i.e., performance at a reduced heart rate, is not dependent on an increased stroke volume, since it takes place before any cardiac enlargement occurs. In this connection we must refer to the section on "Control of Cardiac Function Under Stress," in the section on "The Work of the Heart Under Dynamic Load." According to the findings of Stegemann, (1974), the decreased heart rate in athletes under stress is due to a decrease in sympathetic stimulation. The improved metabolic state of the trained muscle also affects cardiac function via the chemoreceptors. As already mentioned in the discussion on the regulation of the resting frequency, we are probably dealing here also with a feedback mechanism. The increased stroke volume of the athlete's heart provides good perfusion to the muscle, even in the face of a decreased sympathetic drive.

This behavior of the trained heart is analogous to the effect of the *beta blockers*, as pointed out by Roskamm (1972) (Fig 3–16). At rest, and under submaximal load, the athlete's heart works as though it were a heart under the influence of a β-blocker. Under similar load increments, the heart rate and the myocardial *contractility*, as measured by the maximal rate of pressure increase, are both decreased. In effect, the work of the heart must be affected similarly, whether the peripheral sympathetic stimulation is decreased in the athlete's heart, or whether sympathetic stimulation is blocked in the normal heart.

It would be a mistake, however, to place too much weight on this analogy. In contrast to the β-blocked heart, which has only a limited maximal heart rate and contractility, the trained heart still has the maximal heart rate and contractility available to it under conditions of stress. The range of performance of the β-blocked heart is curtailed and that of the trained heart is expanded. For a given increment of stress both the rate and contractility of the β-blocked—and trained—heart are reduced. Looking at the situation under maximal stress conditions,

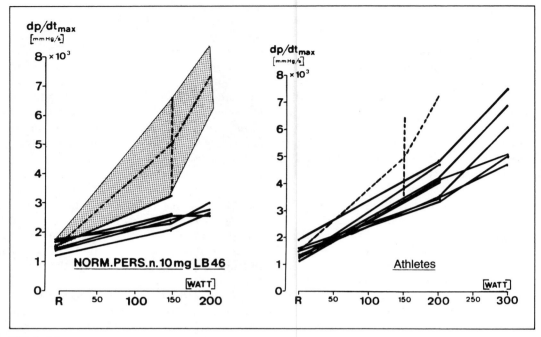

FIG 3–16.

Comparison of the effects of beta blockade *(left)* and physical conditioning *(right)* on contractility under load conditions as measured by the rate of pressure increase in the left ventricle (after Roskamm, 1972). On the left the normal range is indicated by *cross hatching*. The increase in contractility in relation to load is evident. Under beta-blockade there is practically no increase in contractility. On the *right,* these relationships are illustrated in the fully trained endurance athlete. At low levels of load the relationships are similar to those found in the β-blocked person, i.e., the contractility rises only slightly because of the modest sympathetic drive. At higher load levels, maximal contractility is achieved in exactly the same way as in the nontrained person.

however, the *reserves in both rate and contractility* are reduced in the β-blocked heart and increased in the trained heart.

These findings can be substantiated by echocardiography. According to Bubenheimer (1977), the diastolic diameter of the athlete's heart is increased at low stress levels and decreased as the intensity of the stress increases. The noninvasive echocardiographic technique can demonstrate the functional relationships in the athlete's heart just as well as the invasive techniques used by Roskamm (1972). Echocardiography is shown to be an important method in the functional assessment of the athlete's heart.

The behavior of varying functional sizes as determined by echocardiography

in athletes under rest and during exercise is shown in Figure 3–17. A glance at these values should stimulate additional commentary concerning the reliability of echocardiography in measuring stroke volume: It is frequently argued that it is unreliable in giving absolute stroke volume data, but that it is suitable to determine changes in stroke volume in the same subject under different conditions. As seen from the values in Figure 3–17, we found a continuously increasing stroke volume in relationship to the increase in the intensity of stress.

If these results are compared with those found with invasive techniques (see Fig 2–1), it appears that they can not be accurately reproduced. The stroke vol

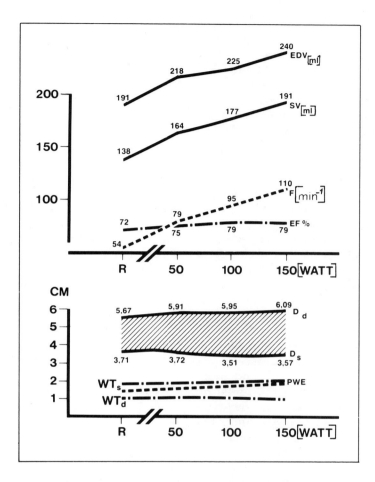

FIG 3–17.
Echocardiographic values obtained by the M-mode technique, under increasing load conditions in athletes in the supine position. The data show a slight increase in the diastolic diameter *(Dₔ)* and a decrease in the systolic diameter *(Dₛ)*. From these data a slight increase in the ejection fraction *(EF)* and a load-dependent increase in the end-diastolic volume *(EDV)* and stroke volume *(SV)* can be calculated, us-*ing the cubic function.* Increasing load causes an increase in the motion of the posterior wall *(PWE)* while the systolic *(WTₛ)* and diastolic *(WTₔ)* wall thickness remains constant. The heart rate is indicated. A comparison with behavior of the stroke volume in Figure 2–1 shows that the load-dependent increase in the stroke volume on the echo does not correspond to the actual events.

ume increases at the beginning of the stress, but then remains relatively constant, independently of the increasing stress conditions. For this reason great caution is indicated in evaluating the stroke volume data obtained in the athlete's heart under stress conditions by the M-mode echocardiographic technique. On the other hand, the values obtained directly from the echocardiogram, and those parameters that do not require com-

plicated calculations, give an excellent opportunity for a noninvasive evaluation of athlete's heart function. These include in addition to the diameter of the left ventricle, the *fractional shortening* (LVED − LVSD/LVED) and the *mean velocity of circumferential fiber-shortening* (VCF = fractional shortening/ejection time).

In concluding the discussion of the function of the athlete's heart, the concept of *economy* must be presented. This concept has undergone a change under the influence of the findings already presented. In the older German literature of the 1950s and 1960s, it is understood primarily quantitatively, in the sense of a decrease in external cardiac work for equal physical performance. Besides a decrease in cardiac output at rest, or under equal stress conditions, it was assumed that there was a decrease in blood pressure under identical performances. Thus, the product of volume and pressure that is generated by the trained heart is clearly less than the product generated by the nontrained heart. The above-demonstrated hemodynamic findings have shown in the meantime, however, that the volume work of the trained heart is not decreased. The same is true for the pressure work. Cross-sectional studies by Reindell (1960) and Hollmann (1976) showed no difference in pressure under similar loads when trained and nontrained hearts were compared. Similar results were obtained when cross-sectional and longitudinal studies were compared using direct arterial pressure measurements (see Fig 2–6).

While the pulse rate is greatly affected by an increase in vagal tone at rest, or by a decrease in sympathetic tone under stress conditions in the trained athlete, this is not true for the volume-work or pressure-work. As already discussed in detail, the cardiac output that is required depends on the specific oxygen requirements, i.e., on the performance that must be achieved and not on the level of training. The peripheral resistance that together with the cardiac output determines the blood pressure at any given time depends on the ratio of contraction versus tension of the musculature, and is also not dependent on the level of training.

It can, therefore, be determined that the "economy" of the trained heart consists less in a decrease in the external work of the heart than in the way in which this work is accomplished. By reducing the sympathetic drive, the rate and contractility decrease. Both reduce the *myocardial oxygen requirements*. Heiss (1976) found a 35% decrease in myocardial oxygen utilization. On the other hand, a prolongation of the diastole prolongs that phase of the cardiac cycle that is important for the perfusion of the heart. The trained heart is therefore distinguished by a reduction in its oxygen requirements under similar loads, and by an improvement in its perfusion characteristics. Since this "economy" is primarily due to a change in the peripheral control, it is not necessarily related to the dimensional adaptations of the athlete's heart. The development of functional adaptation can therefore be seen at a level of training intensity, which does not lead to a hypertrophy of the athlete's heart.

CLINICAL ASPECTS

As already emphasized in the introductory remarks, the clinical interpretation of the athlete's heart presents considerable difficulties by virtue of its size and because of the frequent ECG abnormalities demonstrated by it. On the other hand, consideration must be given to the high stresses to which this heart is exposed during training and during competitions. Even minor cardiac injuries, which would be given only minimal attention in the nontrained, may assume threatening consequences in this situation. In the clinical evaluation it is important therefore to identify those athletes who, because of organic heart disease, are in danger during athletic activity, even though the disease itself may be of a trifling nature. On the other hand, it is important to avoid the pitfall of labeling athletes as cardiac patients just because the adaptation phenomena of the athlete's heart are being misinterpreted.

Electrocardiographic Findings

The experience obtained in a large outpatient, sports-cardiology clinic has shown that the clinical problems associated with athlete's heart were most commonly based on ECG findings. These ECG findings in the athlete's heart can be so dramatic that a colleague was moved to write a letter to the Journal of the American Medical Association, urging that routine ECGs should never be done in athletes, since the findings would cause more harm than good. On the basis of striking but unimportant ECG abnormalities, athletes were advised to desist from any further athletic activity. These findings not infrequently also led to unnecessary and dangerous invasive diagnostic tests (Sheehan, 1973). This sarcastic letter underlines the need for the physician who numbers athletes among his patients to become familiar with the peculiarities of the ECG in the athlete's heart; it did not really mean that ECGs should never be done on athletes.

The most important ECG changes will be briefly presented below. The reader interested in a more detailed discussion is referred to an earlier monograph on the subject (Rost, 1980). It must be emphasized that there are no characteristic changes in the ECG of the athlete's heart. The variations observed are the result of hypertrophy and of an increased vagal tone, which can also be seen under all other conditions that lead to cardiac hypertrophy and to an autonomic imbalance. There are three basic ECG patterns that are of significance in the evaluation of the athlete's heart.

1. *Normal, physiologic variants as the result of training* that can lead to diagnostic difficulties, if the physician is unaware of their incidence in the athlete. As far as the signs of *left ventricular hypertrophy* (increased left ventricular Sokolow-Lyon index) and *right ventricular*

hypertrophy (increased right ventricular Sokolow-Lyon index) are concerned, the reader is referred to the section on "Electrocardiographic Signs of Hypertrophy." An increased vagal tone can lead to arrhythmias and functional conduction disturbances in addition to the training bradycardia. The *arrhythmias* can be either supraventricular or ventricular. The supraventricular arrhythmias are classified according to the location of the P wave. The *coronary sinus rhythm* shows an inverted P wave and a normal conduction time (Fig 3–18). In the *upper nodal rhythm* the conduction time is shortened. In a *middle nodal rhythm* there is no P wave. The *lower nodal rhythm* can be recognized by an inverted P wave, which falls after the ventricular complex. This phenomenon is found only very rarely in the athlete, and so is the *wandering pacemaker*, in which the impulse generation passes from the sinus node to the middle nodal rhythm.

The *simple AV dissociation*, which occurs frequently in the athlete, is often mistakenly identified as a wandering pacemaker. The AV dissociation is characterized by a P wave, which is always upright, but that occurs at varying distances ahead of the ventricular complex (Fig 3–19). We are dealing here with the simplest form of an overlap between two pacemakers (*simple para-arrhythmia*), the sinus node and the AV node, that alternate in assuming control. In contrast to the AV node, the rate of the sinus node is significantly influenced by autonomic and by respiratory effects. If the sinus wave is relatively late, the AV node will fire, and the P wave will fall just before the ventricular complex. This imitates the picture of a shortened conduction time, which, in fact, does not exist. Related to the simple AV dissociation, but extremely rarely found in the athlete, is the *interference-dissociation*. It differs from the simple AV dissociation by the appearance of a retrograde, protective

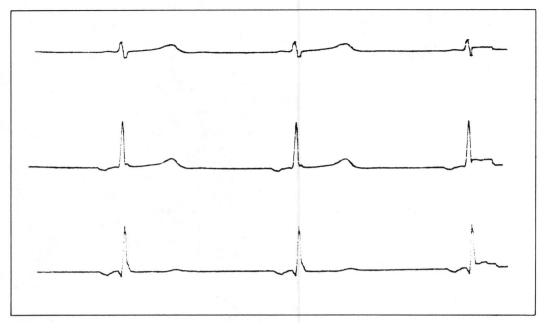

FIG 3–18.
Example of a coronary sinus rhythm in an endurance athlete (standard leads). The coronary sinus rhythm is characterized by negative P waves and a normal conduction time. The ECG is from the same athlete whose heart was shown in Figure 3–2.

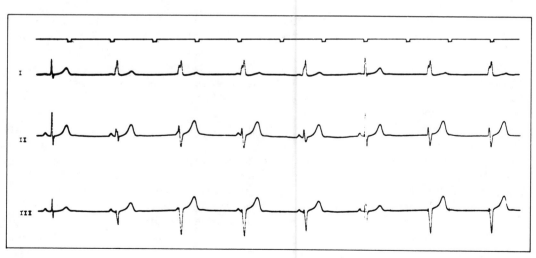

FIG 3–19.
Example of a simple atrioventricular (AV) dissociation with a ventricular escape rhythm. The AV separation appears to be changing. The first ventricular complex is preceded by a normal p wave. The third beat is a ventricular escape beat; the second one is a fusion beat. From the fourth beat onward, the sinus rate is faster than the ventrical escape focus. The sixth beat represents the resumption of control by the sinus node.

block. The impulse originating in the AV node does not lead to a retrograde atrial stimulation. Thus, the P wave is maintained and can "wander" through the entire cardiac cycle. If it falls fairly late, it can again assume control (Fig 3–20). This picture, however, is usually reserved for pathologic conditions, particularly digitalis intoxication. We have seen this phenomenon only very rarely in the several thousand athletes whom we have studied.

Not uncommon, and yet always surprising to the physician unfamiliar with the ECG of the athlete's heart, is the appearance of a ventricular arrhythmia (Fig 3–21). Such ECG tracings are frequently mistaken for an intermittent bundle-branch block or for an intermittent Wolff-Parkinson-White syndrome. This error can be avoided by realizing that the widened ventricular complex is not preceded by a P wave. If such a ventricular arrhythmia is combined with a simple AV dissociation, the picture of an apparent "alternating axis deviation" can be seen, because of the fusion of the atrial and ventricular beats. This is not uncommon in the athlete's heart ECG (Fig 3–22).

It is well known that as far as functional conduction disturbances are concerned, prolongation of the conduction time (first degree AV block, second degree, Wenckebach type AV block), can occur in athletes. The prolongation of the conduction time is usually slight, and the PQ interval rarely exceeds 0.22 seconds. Significant first degree AV blocks are extremely rare. While the Wenckebach periodicity is extremely rare in the non-trained person, according to the literature, it appears in the ECG tracing of the athlete in about 0.5% to 1% of all cases (Fig 3–23).

By Holter monitoring even the sleep ECG, we found a second degree AV block

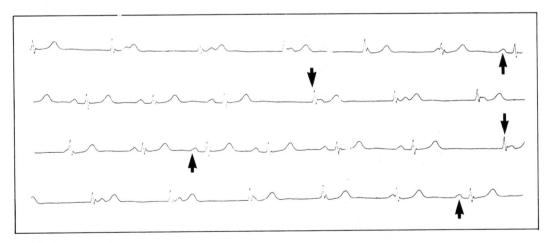

FIG 3–20.
Example of an interference-disassociation in an athlete. The continuous strip recording illustrates the mechanism of this rhythm disturbance. The upper strip starts with a supraventricular rhythm originating in a parasystolic focus. In contrast to the simple pararhythm, this rhythm is characterized by a retrograde block, i.e., the stimulus is not transmitted in a retrograde fashion to the atria, so that the p waves are not extinguished and may fall even after the ventricular complex. The respiratory arrhythmia causes the sinus node to become faster than the escape focus. The p waves are separated from the ventricular complexes and are finally in a lead position in the last complex of the upper strip (captured beat). With the respiratory slowing of the sinus rhythm, the parasystolic focus again assumes the lead in the third complex of the second strip and the sequence is repeated in a cyclical fashion. The *arrows* pointing up indicate the point where the sinus node takes over the leading function, while the points where the escape focus takes over are indicated by the *arrows* pointing down.

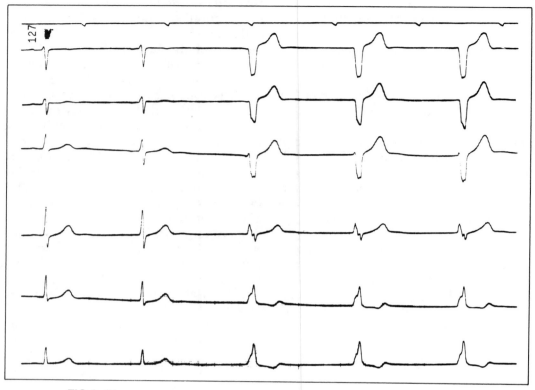

FIG 3–21.
Example of a ventricular escape rhythm in an athlete recorded from chest leads.
The escape rhythm starts with the third beat.

in 10% of all the athletes studied (Horst, 1983). Although this was denied for a long time, even *third degree heart blocks,* of a purely functional nature, can be seen in athletes. Venerando (1979) described two well-documented cases of this finding. We studied a female long-distance runner whose ECG showed periodic total AV dissociation (Fig 3–24). Further study, including a bundle of His ECG, failed to show any organic cardiac disease.

The question as to whether there is such a thing as a purely functional *sino-atrial block* (SA block) in the athlete was answered in the negative in most parts of the literature. On the other hand, it is difficult to see why increased vagal tone should be unable to produce an AV block, but not an SA block. We have seen

ECG changes in the trained person, which could be formally interpreted as SA blocks, even though it was difficult to decide in the individual cases whether or not we were dealing with an extreme case of *respiratory arrhythmia.* If, however, such changes appear in conjunction with stress (Fig 3–25), they cannot be interpreted as respiratory arrhythmia.

The functional nature of these impulse-generating and conduction disturbances can be recognized by the fact that they disappear immediately under exercise. On the other hand, it may be true here also, as already discussed in connection with bradycardia, that even functional impulse-generation disturbances may become clinically relevant if they are superimposed upon a damaged conduction system.

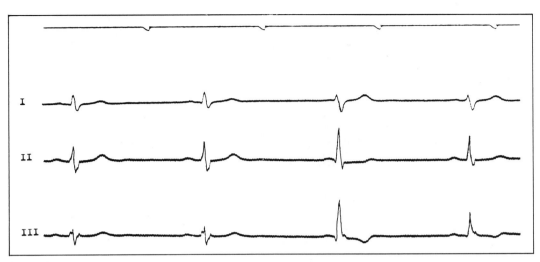

FIG 3–22.
Example of an apparent change in dominance. From the third beat on the standard leads, the type changes from a *left dominance* to a *right dominance*. The PR interval changes at the same time. This shows that this is a simple *para-arrhythmia* where the third beat originates from an escape focus and the fourth beat is again a fusion beat.

2. *ECG changes that are due to physical conditioning and which cannot be distinguished from pathologic phenomena* on the basis of their configuration. These can be seen primarily in the area of repolarization. They consist of ST segment depression or elevation, and T-wave inversion, which can be mistaken on the ECG for epicardial injury as seen in pericarditis, or even for a myocardial infarction (Figs 3–26 and 3–27). These changes are so striking and occur so frequently in athletes that they appear regularly in the literature (Rost, 1980). Only a brief discussion of these changes will be presented. First of all, it must be emphasized that these *repolarization changes* are not limited to "athletics." Even though they do occur relatively frequently in athletes, they do occur also in the nontrained person, in children, young people, women, and blacks. There is no uniform explanation for these phenomena in athletes. Some authors, particularly Butschenko (1967) and Plas (1974), insist that these are not physiologic variants. On the other hand, long-range studies by Venerando, (1979) in 52 athletes who showed these changes, failed to reveal the development of any pathologic changes. There is no instance in the literature where invasive diagnostic techniques, even coronary arteriography, showed any organic heart disease. It is true that Frick (1975) did have one patient, an athlete, who did show these findings on ECG, and in whom noninvasive diagnostic techniques, i.e., echocardiography and myocardial scintigraphy, did reveal evidence of myocardial damage. This case, however, was not typical, since the athlete did complain of cardiac symptoms. On the other hand, it must be stressed that in the series of athletes studied by Maron (1980) and who died suddenly from a hypertrophic cardiomyopathy, there was one athlete who did show similar ECG changes.

On the basis of these facts it would be a mistake to either minimize or dramatize these ECG findings. They obviously can occur in the trained heart without being based on any demonstrable pathology.

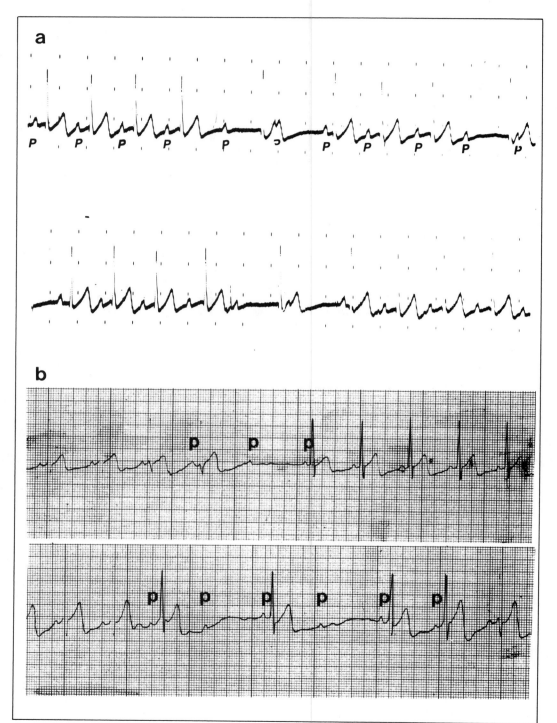

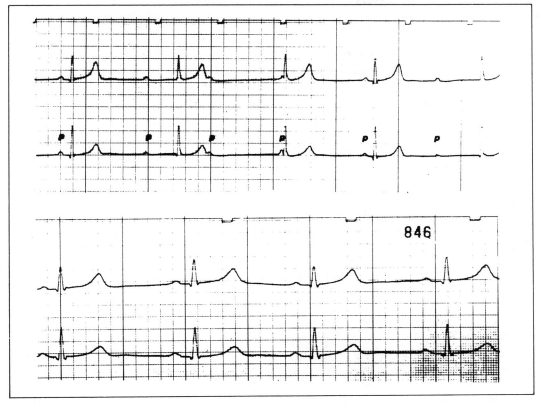

FIG 3–24.

Example of a functionally induced, third-degree atrioventricular disassociation in a female long-distance runner. This change occurred briefly in a switch from a Wenckeback periodicity. Under load the block dis-

appeared immediately *(below)*. The leads are standard leads I and II and the paper speed is 85 mm/seconds above and 50 mm/seconds below.

The etiology is totally unclear. Hypertrophy was blamed and so was an increased vagal tone and electrolyte abnormalities. None of these could be documented. The observation that they occurred more frequently in blacks led to the suggestion that they were race-related (Littmann, 1946), even though they do occur in white athletes as well. The observation made by Venerando, that these changes frequently disappear on the stress ECG, suggests that they may be functional. Yet, we have seen cases where such ST segment changes appeared only on the stress

FIG 3–23.

Example of a second degree atrioventricular block in athletes. **a,** a typical Wenckebach periodicity in a 12-year-old swimmer. The p waves are pronounced and show the characteristic increase in the PR interval. The sixth p wave is no longer transmitted and with the seventh p wave the Wenckebach period begins again. **b,** in comparison, shows a Mobitz type II. The PR intervals remain the same but in the *upper* part there is a single instance of no transmission. In the *lower* part this occurs for a short period as part of a 2:1 block. While the Wenckebach periodicity is considered normal in the performance athletes, the Mobitz type is not. The second tracing was obtained by Holter monitoring from an athlete in whom very thorough studies, including a bundle of His electrocardiogram, failed to show any cardiac damage.

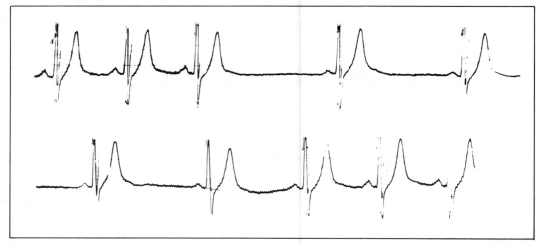

FIG 3–25.

Example of a sinoatrial block during the first minute after exercise in a swimmer. After the third beat the individual p waves coincide with the ventricular com-plexes. After the eighth beat a normal relationship is reestablished.

ECG. The example shown in Figure 3–27 suggests the importance of a hyper-trophic component, since the repolariza-tion disturbances appeared during an ex-tremely high level of training, and disappeared after the training was dis-continued. Yet again, such changes are found even in the moderately trained ath-lete as well.

It would be totally wrong, therefore, to label athletes who show these ECG changes as cardiac patients. We have seen many athletes who wound up in a coronary care unit with the tentative di-agnosis of a myocardial infarct. This can be illustrated by the following, striking example: We were presented with a 42-year-old marathon runner who was said to have suffered a myocardial infarct for an evaluation for cardiac rehabilitation.

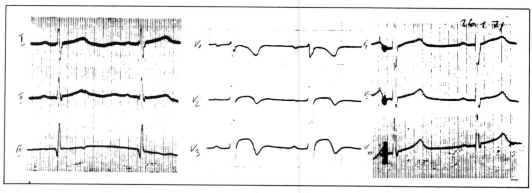

FIG 3–26.

An example of a significant repolarization distur-bance in an athlete. The electrocardiogram was sub-mitted to us by a general practitioner because of its peculiar configuration. The thorough cardiologic work-up and a 10-year follow-up failed to reveal any cardiac pathology. The change consists of ST seg-ment elevation and transiently inverted T waves mostly in the V_2 and V_3 leads.

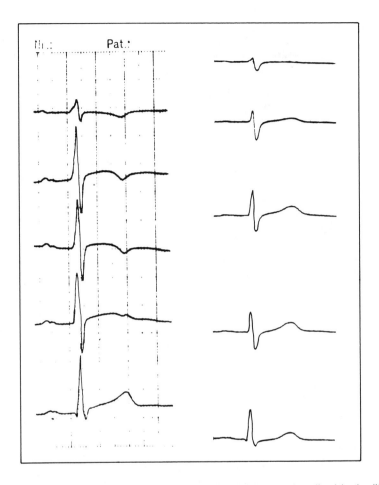

FIG 3–27.

The electrocardiogram shows repolarization disturbances similar to those in Figure 3–26, although in a
less-pronounced form. The tracing on the left was obtained from a bicycle racer who had the largest cardiac volume ever described in the literature. Follow-
up studies 12 years later showed a disappearance of
these changes.

At a routine examination in the absence
of any complaints, he was found to have
an ST segment elevation, on the left precordial leads, with a transition to a pre-
terminal T wave. At the same time his
enzymes were elevated: serum glutamic-
oxaloacetic transaminase to 37 and crea-
tine phosphokinase to 110 milliunits/ml.
Even though the athlete insisted that he
was feeling perfectly fine and had run 20
km the day before, he was admitted to a
coronary care unit with the diagnosis of a
silent infarction, and was kept flat on his
back for 3 weeks.

The diagnosis of an infarction in this
case was clearly an error. These types of
ECG changes do occur in athletes. The
enzyme elevations can be explained on
the basis of the long-distance run. This
case history illustrates the difficulties
that can be encountered when examining
athletes. On the other hand, it would be
equally wrong to assume that all such
changes are harmless, since athletes obviously can also suffer from heart disease. A thorough clinical evaluation is required. These should be based in most
cases on noninvasive techniques. As

stated above, invasive studies are usually not indicated. The following measures have been proved to be particularly important.

    A. Review earlier ECG tracings, since the same changes can be observed in the same athlete at different times.

    B. Obtain a stress ECG. This may seem a dubious practice to a clinician who sees a tracing like the one shown in Figure 3–26. Nevertheless, we must realize that we are dealing with symptom-free young men who are frequently and severely stressed on the athletic field. The disappearance of the findings under stress would constitute an important point.

    C. Obtain an ECG after an oral potassium loading.

    D. Obtain an ultrasound cardiogram to rule out a hypertrophic cardiomyopathy. If possible, this should be a two-dimensional representation, since a unidimensional representation may miss a localized lesion.

Naturally, careful cardiac surveillance and monitoring are essential. Initially the athlete should be advised to abandon any significant conditioning stress or competitive activity until it can be assumed with some assurance several months later that there is no organic heart disease present or in a stage of development.

3. *ECG changes outside the physiologic range* cannot be discussed here in detail, since all possible ECG changes occur in the athlete as well. Only the most important problems can be mentioned here that are likely to occur in the practice of sports cardiology. It must again be emphasized that even minor ECG changes, which would be ignored in the nontrained person, may assume great importance under the heavy stress conditions of the athlete's heart. In sports cardiology the apparently minor problems cause the greatest headaches for the physician. Usually there is no question that an athlete with a complete, organic AV block or a complete left bundle-branch block should be forbidden to continue high endurance physical exercise. In contrast, a complete right bundle-branch block is usually considered to be relatively harmless in the nontrained person. Can this be tolerated in the endurance-conditioned athlete? If single premature beats are considered harmless, how many can be tolerated in athletes: 2, 5, or 20 per minute?

Paroxysmal tachycardia is usually considered to be relatively meaningless in young people without organic heart disease. How must it be viewed in the high performance athlete, when one considers that under conditions of extreme acidosis, even mild tachycardias can trigger a ventricular fibrillation? For example, there are 400-meter runners who have a pH of 6.8 after the race. Keren (1981) pointed out that fatal accidents occurred in athletes with Wolff-Parkinson-White syndrome, probably triggered by a tachycardia. For this reason, high performance athletes who are severely stressed during their athletic events should be forbidden to continue if they show such tachycardias. Unfortunately this can have serious economic repercussions, particularly in the professional athlete. In such instances it may be very difficult for the sports-cardiologist to find the middle road between the demands of athletic, medical, and economic considerations. Even though medical considerations must be given absolute priority, the athlete should not be made to suffer from medical *"over protection."*

In this connection, the most important ECG phenomena should be considered as follows.

According to a frequently-held view, *premature contractions* occur more frequently in the athlete than in the nontrained person because of the increased resting vagal tone in the former. We found premature beats in only 0.6% of the routine ECGs obtained from athletes. In 18-hour Holter monitoring, of course, the incidence was much higher. At rest, an incidence of 26% was found by both Horst (1983) and ourselves. If we add the premature beats that occurred under stress conditions, we found that 42% of the 50 endurance athletes studied had a significant incidence of premature beats. Holter monitoring showed the appearance of pronounced "runs" of the Lown type IVb ventricular beats in three athletes at rest. The premature beats appearing under stress conditions, however, were always single and rare.

Conversely, neither routine ECG tracings nor Holter monitoring shows more premature beats in the athletes than in the nontrained person. Comparable studies in nontrained young people are unfortunately rare. The best source is the study of Brodsky (1977), who found premature beats in 55% of his subjects under Holter monitoring. His data are of somewhat limited value, since some of his subjects must have been at least partially trained. When we restricted our findings to the athletes with a resting bradycardia of less than 45 beats per minute, we did not observe an increased incidence of premature beats. This further supports the assumption that the increased vagal tone in the trained athlete contributes little to the development of premature beats (Table 3–2).

A particularly difficult problem is presented by the appearance of potentially dangerous runs of premature beats in apparently healthy endurance athletes (Fig 3–28). This problem is not specific to

TABLE 3-2.

Summary of Findings Obtained on 18-Hour Monitoring of 50 German Championship Class Endurance Athletes*

	AT REST	UNDER LOAD
PREMATURE BEATS (EB)		
Single supraventricular EB	6	5
Runs of supraventricular EB	2	–
Single ventricular EB	4	5
Runs of ventricular EB	1	–
Total	13 (26%)	10 (20%)
	42%	
OTHER ARRHYTHMIAS		
Para-arrhythmia	3	–
Escape rhythm	1	–
SA block	1	–
AV block 1st degree	1	–
AV block 2nd degree	5	–

EXTREME BRADYCARDIA (SLEEP)/TACHYCARDIA (EXERCISE)

<30/min	0	<180/min	11
30–39/min	12	180–200/min	24
40–49/min	31	201–210/min	14
50–59/min	7	>210/min	1

*The studies were performed on long-distance runners, bicycle racers, and cross-country skiers, by Horst (1983). Each study period included a minimum of a 1-hour exercise period and also a period of sleep.

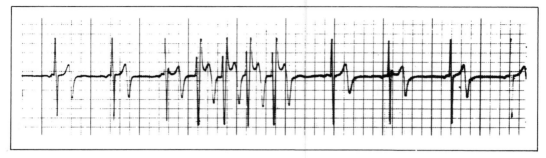

FIG 3–28.
Incidental finding of a run of premature beats during Holter monitoring in a completely healthy athlete. The observation was made by Horst (1983) and is in the files of our institute.

athletes, since such findings can occasionally be seen in the nontrained person without any demonstrable cardiac disease. As far as the literature is concerned, reference must be made to the review article by Meinertz (1983). The basic problem is really one of interpretation. The American literature frequently refers to "healthy patients," since no organic heart disease can be demonstrated in them. The recommendation is made to play down the importance of these findings. The currently available, long-term observations are not sufficient to state positively that in the absence of organic heart findings, such disturbances in rhythm can be held responsible for any of the always devastating sudden deaths in young people. On the other hand, in the absence of positive autopsy findings, ventricular fibrillation caused by such rhythm disturbances cannot be excluded.

Complex arrhythmias of this type cannot, however, be held responsible for the sudden death of an athlete actually engaged in exercise, since the arrhythmias seem to appear only at rest. In the present state of our knowledge, it does not seem to be appropriate to forbid further athletic activity purely on the basis of such findings. This is particularly true when one considers that, according to the above discussion, the training-dependent adaptation phenomena of the heart do not facilitate the appearance of such arrhythmias. Another question concerns the potential, long-term antiarrhythmic prophylactic therapy in athletes with such findings. In this situation we must weigh the relative hazards of the arrhythmia versus the side effects of the medication. In any case, if the decision is made to treat the athlete pharmacologically, further athletic activity should be discouraged in view of the cardiodepressant side effects of the antiarrhythmic drugs. These problems will be further discussed below, in connection with paroxysmal tachycardia and in the section on "Physical Exercise and Cardiac Medications."

The fresh appearance of premature beats in an athlete should always be taken seriously, since they may be an indication of a developing carditis. In such cases it is critical to search for evidence of a focal infection. Appropriate therapy of dental abscesses or tonsillitis has frequently led to the disappearance of such arrhythmias. The appearance of premature beats in the athlete under stress conditions is frequently related to infections. In view of the very heavy stress imposed on athletes, it is much more difficult to evaluate premature beats in these persons than in the nontrained individual. If premature beats are present all the time, it can be assumed that they are not due to an acute disease process, but to myocardial scarring or to a "reentry" problem. In this case they must be evaluated on the basis of their shape and their incidence. If they are multifocal, or appear in runs or clearly increase in numbers under stress, further athletic activity should be discouraged.

Paroxysmal tachycardias must be evaluated on the basis of their frequency and their configuration. If they are triggered relatively frequently by physical exercise, high performance athletics should be forbidden. It would certainly be desirable to record the arrhythmia. The attacks are frequently triggered, at least to some extent, by sports-related physical exercise. Apparently there are some mechanical factors here, such as the physical agitation of the heart under certain athletic maneuvers, that may have major significance. Stress testing will usually not reproduce them. If they occur relatively frequently, an attempt should be made to record them by Holter monitoring. Very high frequencies and arrhythmias within the framework of the tachycardia, or a very frequent occurrence, should be sufficient cause to advise against any further athletic activity.

The same is true for certain forms of activity, where the occurrence of such a tachycardia may seriously endanger the athlete, e.g., diving, flying, etc. Under no circumstances should the athlete be made "fit to perform" with antiarrhythmic medications. Almost all available antiarrhythmic drugs are negative inotropes. If under such treatment some untoward event should occur during an athletic event, it will be impossible to decide whether this was due to the arrhythmia, or to the therapy. It should be a fundamental tenet that an athlete who requires drug therapy because of the seriousness of the cardiac condition should not participate in high performance athletics. The situation could be quite different in mass sports.

Paroxysmal tachycardias must play a central role in connection with the evaluation of *Wolff-Parkinson-White syndrome* in athletes. This syndrome has quite particular significance for the athlete's heart for the following reasons.

A. The pre-excitation syndrome is considered to occur more frequently in the athlete than in the nontrained person. According to our own observations, Wolff-Parkinson-White syndrome occurs in athletes slightly more frequently than in the average population. The average figures are, however, obtained from the general population. Since Wolff-Parkinson-White syndrome is somewhat more frequent in young people, it is possible that the somewhat higher incidence in athletes is due to the fact that athletes belong to this subset of the population, and not due to their level of physical conditioning.

B. Wolff-Parkinson-White syndrome is frequently misread on the ECG tracing. Accordingly, the wrong diagnosis is frequently made in athletes with the Wolff-Parkinson-White syndrome. This happens particularly when the physician does not realize that in patients with Wolff-Parkinson-White syndrome, stress ECGs frequently show false repolarization disturbances.

C. The frequent appearance of tachycardias in the athlete raises all the problems already discussed above.

Although the literature occasionally mentions the Wolff-Parkinson-White syndrome as the reason for forbidding high performance athletics, it can be assumed that they were dealing with an "abnormality" of the ECG pattern only, provided that there was no tachycardia and that Wolff-Parkinson-White syndrome was not a sign of organic heart disease.

Deaths, in connection with paroxysmal tachycardia and Wolff-Parkinson-White syndrome in athletics, were described in the same way as deaths and Wolff-Parkinson-White syndrome in patients with organic heart disease. Among the athletes who died suddenly with hypertrophic cardiomyopathy described by Maron (1981), there was one who had Wolff-Parkinson-White syndrome. Schmid (1981) describes an athlete who had a Wolff-Parkinson-White tachycardia, and who suffered a fatal myocardial infarct while windsurfing.

It is well known that such changes occur with increased frequency in patients with congenital or acquired heart disease. If these diseases can be excluded and if a careful and complete history fails to reveal any tachycardia, the athlete showing these signs should be allowed to continue his athletic activities.

It must be emphasized, however, that there are many athletes, particularly professional athletes, who are well aware of the potential problems when they first notice the appearance of a tachycardia. For this reason they frequently deny its existence. If the appearance of the tachycardia is known, the evaluation of the tachycardia must take into serious consideration the statements made above. In Wolff-Parkinson-White syndrome, the tachycardia may present as an atrial fibrillation, leading to ventricular fibrillation if there is a 1:1 transmission. Younger athletes with Wolff-Parkinson-White syndrome must be cautioned particularly that serious attacks may only appear later. A 9- or 10-year-old who shows Wolff-Parkinson-White syndrome should avoid sports that require major effort and that in this particular relationship may be very questionable. This youngster should prefer activities such as "play-sports" where the possibility of substitutions makes the appearance of tachycardias much less of a problem.

Among the *conduction defects*, a *complete right bundle-branch block* is seen occasionally among athletes. Even though, and in contrast to the incomplete right bundle-branch block, this can never be considered a physiologic variant, it does appear to be a manifestation of a mild cardiac injury, such as a pericarditis in early childhood. Thus, forbidding all further athletics may not be indicated. Obviously, underlying pathology, particularly an atrial septal defect, must be eliminated. A *complete left bundle-branch block* is also always a pathologic manifestation. We have never yet found a high-performance athlete in whom this ECG change was encountered as an incidental finding. This block should be sufficient reason to advise against any further athletic activity that requires significant physical stress.

Concerning the conduction disturbances between atrium and ventricle, we wish to refer to the functional variants discussed above. A *first degree AV block,* which disappears under stress, should be considered to be physiologic. The same block, if it first appears under stress, must be considered as pathologic. Among the *second degree AV blocks,* the Mobitz type II is always considered to be pathologic, in contrast to the Wenckebach periodicity. Quite recently we observed an athlete with this condition who complained of dizzy spells (see Fig 3–23,B). The bundle of His ECG was unremarkable. Since we occasionally see this type of tracing during Holter monitoring as an incidental finding, it seems that this also may be regarded as a physiologic variant. A *third degree AV block* of organic origin is obviously a contraindication for further high-performance athletics. It is nevertheless amazing how many reserves the heart has in the presence of a congenital AV block. We know of a high-performance soccer player who suffered from a total AV dissociation that was compensated for by a secondary supraventricular center, which under stress could generate a rate of 150 beats per minute. There are also, of course, some grotesque cases, as the one illustrated in Figure 3–29. It represents a female student, who, in spite of a known total AV block, enrolled in physical education. Even after moderate stress, the rate increase was insufficient and worrisome premature beats appeared on the exercise ECG. Obviously such cases represent an absolute contraindication for all types of performance athletics.

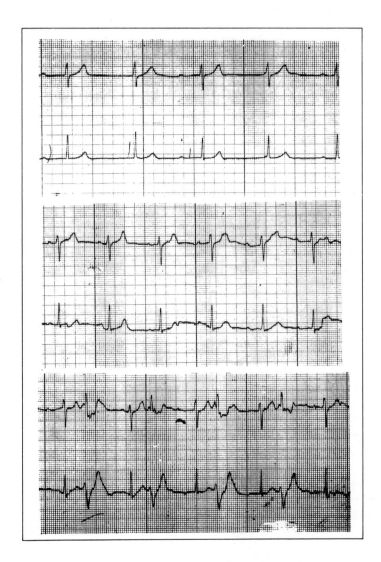

FIG 3–29.

Finding of a complete atrioventricular (AV) block in a female physical education student at the German Sports High School, Cologne. The complete AV block is not seen well on the resting electrocardiogram *(upper tracing)* but is recognizable on closer examination. This student engaged in the physical education curriculum against the strong advice of the University Clinic. Moderate exercise on the bicycle ergometer *(middle tracing)* leads first to an increase in rate of the supraventricular escape focus. With higher loads *(lower tracing)* bigeminal premature beats appear. She was advised to discontinue her physical education studies.

Echocardiographic Findings

Echocardiography has proved useful in sports cardiology, not only as an important tool in the understanding of the functional aspects of the athlete's heart, but it has also opened up new diagnostic avenues. The athlete's heart comes to the physician's attention not only because of its size and its ECG findings, but frequently also because of murmurs, which cannot always be classified as functional. In view of the heavy stress to which the athlete's heart is exposed, it is particularly important to perform exhaustive diagnostic studies. On the other hand, these diagnostic studies should only rarely be invasive, since they rarely lead to surgical intervention. Generally, invasive investigations are not justified merely to come to a definitive decision concerning the continuation of athletic activities. The possibility to assess valvular function through echocardiography is particularly significant, although the limitations of the technique must be kept in mind, particularly in the evaluation of juvenile aortic stenosis.

In addition, the introduction of the ultrasound diagnostic techniques has popularized two cardiac diseases that can be considered to be "ultrasound specific." These are hypertrophic cardiomyopathy, and mitral valve prolapse. In reference to sports-cardiology, two questions must be raised:

1. Since both of these conditions are seen primarily in young people, the question is: how often do they occur in athletes?

2. Can physical conditioning lead to the development of these conditions?

Roeske (1979) had pointed out that an *asymmetrical septal hypertrophy* could be found fairly frequently in athletes who had no apparent organic disease. He found that in 10% of the athletes studied the relationship between the thickness of the septum and the posterior wall exceeded the permissible range of 1.3. We have also seen such cases (see Fig 3–10), but the incidence was lower (3.3%) than Roeske's. These data were published in a comprehensive monograph (Rost, 1982). The incidence depends on the diagnostic technique used. Dickhuth (1979) reports an average value for the septum-posterior wall ratio in runners of 1.27, which means that in a large number of the athletes examined by him, this value was over 1.3. It is also true, however, that in his control group, consisting of nontrained, matched controls, the ratio was quite similar.

According to our experience, a value greater than 1.3 for the septum-posterior wall ratio is frequently due to a thin posterior wall. In the cases of asymmetric septal hypertrophy observed by us, there was no instance of *hypertrophic cardiomyopathy*, or of a systolic anterior movement of the anterior mitral valve leaflet, or of decreased mobility of the septum. So far we have been unable to demonstrate a single, clinically incontrovertible case of cardiomyopathy in at least 1,000 athletes studied by echocardiography. On the other hand, the occurrence of a thickened septum in athletes does raise the question of whether physiologic hypertrophy can progress to a pathologic one, and whether this possibility exists in athletes who may have a congenital tendency for this condition. This interesting question has not to date been pursued in the literature.

In practice then, it can be maintained that septal thickening does occur in athletes, particularly those who engage in the physically most demanding sports. The meaning of these changes is still not clear. There is no convincing evidence to date that these changes can lead to a hypertrophic cardiomyopathy. On this basis, it would seem to be unjustified at this time to forbid further athletic activity for these athletes. On the other hand, a careful cardiac evaluation is indicated. Although already mentioned earlier, it must be emphasized again that, according to the findings of Maron (1980), hypertrophic cardiomyopathy is among the most frequent causes of sudden death in apparently healthy athletes. If in athletically active persons, the clear diagnosis of a pathologic cardiac hypertrophy is made, all forms of athletic activity which are known to lead to further cardiac enlargement should be forbidden. These include all endurance sports and all high performance sports. Play-sports may be allowed to continue on the basis of individual assessment.

The discovery of a *mitral valve prolapse* frequently creates problems in a sports-medicine clinic. We are frequently presented with athletes who are symptom free, but in whom a routine echocardiogram discovered such a state of affairs. The question usually asked in this connection is: should further participation in athletic activities be forbidden? In resolving this question, the following points should be considered: The incidence of mitral prolapse in an obviously healthy population is not well defined. It varies from 1% to 21% depending on the criteria set by the investigator (Heni, 1980; Rettig, 1978). The incidence of 6.9% found by the first author in athletes is well within this range. In our experience, pronounced mitral valve prolapse in an athlete as illustrated in Figure 3–30, is relatively rare.

The significance of a mitral valve prolapse is not known. There are at least two totally contradictory theories as to its origin. One theory claims that this phenomenon was purely valvular in nature and was due to a myxomatous change in the leaflets (McKay, 1973). The other theory claims that this was a functional myocardial disturbance, or to some extent, a peculiar form of cardiomyopathy (Gulotta, 1974). If the second hypothesis is correct, it would probably be a mistake to allow athletes with these findings to continue

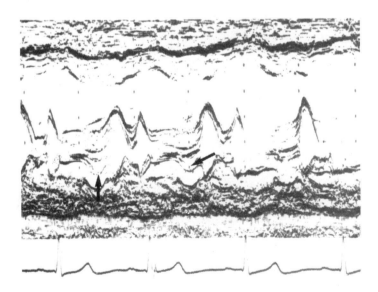

FIG 3–30.
Example of an obvious late systolic mitral valve prolapse during a routine study on a German championship class canoe racer. The *arrow* points to the prolapse of the posterior mitral leaflet. This athlete was followed by us for years and never had any problems related to the high-performance athletic activity.

to participate in any high performance athletic activity.

It is also true, however, that when hemodynamic stress studies were performed in subjects with echocardiographically proven mitral prolapse, substantiated by auscultation, no disturbance in the pump function could be demonstrated (Markworth, 1980). We therefore see no difficulty in allowing athletes to continue their activities if the prolapse is purely an incidental finding on echocardiography. The possibility of significant arrhythmias must, however, be considered in connection with mitral prolapse. For this reason no athletes should be given a "green light" to continue their athletic activities in an area of high-performance athletics in the presence of an ultrasound diagnosis of prolapse, unless the likelihood of arrhythmias has been eliminated by stress ECG and Holter monitoring. To date no death has been reported in connection with this anomaly. There was one athlete in the series reported by Maron (1980) who died suddenly and who did have mitral prolapse. The cause of death, however, was questionable, since this same person also had other cardiac pathology, including a left-sided hypertrophy and dysplastic coronary arteries. When considering the possibility that training may contribute to the development of mitral prolapse, there is the theoretical possibility that after the cessation of the athletic activity and the ensuing regression of the physiologic heart muscle hypertrophy, the valve leaflets become relatively too large and develop a tendency to prolapse. So far there is no evidence whatsoever either for or against this hypothesis.

4

Sport-Related Risk for the Heart

In no case in which death occurred in connection with physical exertion was the subject found at autopsy to be free of a serious disease.

Jokl, 1971

THE NONTRAUMATIC CARDIAC INJURIES

Athletic activity, as Carl Diem has emphasized, is not only a fun-filled, aimless activity that has some positive health benefits, but in addition, it is also a source of significant health hazards. Admittedly, these hazards consisted primarily of lacerations and of orthopedic injuries. Cardiac incidents are relatively rare in athletics. Nevertheless, the sudden death of a young, healthy athlete, or of an older, physically active person, while engaged in athletic activity, is the most dramatic and for those present the most devastating athletic incident. In such instances it is impossible to avoid the question of whether the affected person might not be still alive if he had not engaged in athletics, which he probably did for the sake of his health.

If there is a cardiac incident, e.g., sudden death or myocardial infarction, that takes place during athletic activity,

in each instance the question must be asked if whether or not there is a causal relationship between the physical activity and the cardiac incident. Since most people, including physicians, have a deep-seated need for explanations, such a causal relationship is almost always assumed. But, on the other hand, since such incidents occur during rest as well, the question must be raised of whether the cardiac incident occurred *during* athletic activity or *because of* athletic activity.

The following questions must be answered.

1. Does physical activity, by itself, increase the risk of cardiac incidents?

2. If the answer to the first question is in the affirmative, is this true only for the already-injured heart, or for the healthy heart as well?

3. Does the hypertrophy and increased vagal tone of the athlete's heart increase this risk for the athlete at rest and/or during physical exercise?

Only epidemiologic studies can find an answer to these questions. It must be emphasized at this point that the currently available epidemiologic data are insufficient to give a conclusive answer in this matter. This is partly due to the fact that such cardiac incidents are relatively rare, at least in the healthy, young athlete. The first question that must thus be answered is: how often do such incidents occur in athletics?

We have figures only for those athletic cardiac incidents that have resulted in sudden death. We have no statistics for any other type of cardiac incident. The frequency of sudden death in athletics varies considerably from report to report.

According to a statement of the German Athletic Association, the Sports Association Insurance Company reported 187 deaths in 1981 in connection with athletic activity. Sixty-two of these deaths were apparently due to accidents. The remaining 125 were listed as "incidental deaths" and thus were considered to be more or less incidental to the athletic activity. If one assumes that the percentage of the general population that participates in athletics outside of the athletic associations is approximately the same as the percentage that constitutes the membership of the athletic associations, the total number of athletic-related deaths in West Germany must be put at 350 to 400 per year. Such estimates are naturally very unsatisfactory, particularly when one considers that the age and health conditions of those engaged in athletics outside of the associations is likely to be less satisfactory than those of the predominantly younger members of the associations.

A careful analysis of all the sports-related deaths in the German Federal Republic in the years 1966 to 1975, comprising a total of 124 cases, was reported by Munschek (1977). Twenty-eight of these cases were due to trauma, and 77 were due to organ pathology. Sixty-seven of the deaths were due to cardiac causes: 59 were due to coronary artery disease and eight to myocarditis. Based on these figures, it can be stated that every other athletic-related death is due to cardiac causes, and that each year about 200 people die a cardiac death during athletic activity in the German Federal Republic.

In this connection, the most important question is whether these are "incidental deaths," i.e., really coincidental events, that might have taken place at any time, and anywhere, or whether physical activity increased the risk of sudden cardiac death. In this matter reference must be made to the exhaustive studies by Moritz and Zamcheck, who reviewed 40,000 autopsy protocols in the U.S. Army between 1942 and 1946. There were 98 sudden cardiac deaths in this group, of whose physical activity at the time of death, information was available. According to these statistics, the soldiers who died suddenly spent 33% of their time sleeping and 17% of their time in vigorous physical exercise. Fifteen percent of the deaths occurred during sleep and 29% during major physical effort. These numbers suggest that in the event of preexisting heart disease, particularly coronary artery disease, physical activity is a possible trigger mechanism for the sudden death.

On the other hand, these authors found no statistical relationship between sudden death and the level of physical activity in 127 soldiers who died suddenly, but in whom the autopsy did not reveal any specific cause of death. If one assumes that the cause of death in the majority of these cases had to be a ventricular fibrillation, the etiology of which could not be established in a retrospective fashion, it can be stated that physical stress can trigger sudden death in the previously injured heart, but that it was an accidental occurrence in the healthy heart. Since half of the athletic deaths could be attributed to a preexisting organic heart lesion, these cannot be regarded as "incidental" deaths, i.e., being purely due to chance.

Friedman (1973) reaches the same conclusion and points out that the instantaneous cardiac death is almost always due to ventricular fibrillation, and occurs much more frequently under severe or even moderate physical activity.

This statement is based on the data obtained from 59 coronary artery patients who died suddenly. More than half of them died either during, or immediately following, physical exercise. This pronounced relationship between instantaneous death and physical activity is substantiated by a Finnish study by Vuori (1978). This author, in a very well-known study, analyzed 2,606 sudden deaths that occurred in Finland in 1 year, and for which an autopsy protocol was available. If only those deaths were considered that occurred within 30 seconds, almost all of them were associated with physical activity.

Friedman therefore reaches the conclusion that the instantaneous death in the postinfarction patient is not due to another infarct, but to an electrically-induced cardiac arrest, which occurs in a chronically and severely ill heart. On the basis of this observation the author asks the critical question: "Whether it is worth risking an instantaneous coronary death by indulging in an activity the possible benefit of which to the human coronary vasculature has yet to be proved." His question of whether or not it is possible that we may have forgotten that it is the coronary vasculature, not the myocardium, that needs our enthusiastic prophylaxis or therapy, may seem heretical to some of the devoted supporters of the exercise therapy in coronary heart disease but may also make them think.

On the other hand, no undue weight should be placed on such numbers or observations. The estimate of 300 to 400 annual deaths during physical activity becomes negligible when we compare it with the 700,000 citizens who die annually in the German Federal Republic. It would never do to bad-mouth the positive health benefits of athletics on the basis of the exceptionally rare fatality. According to a statistical study by Jung (1982) in Nordrhein-Westfalen, there was one death that occurred because of or during athletic activity per 75,000 athletes among the members of the organized athletic associations. The obvious conclusion is drawn by Friedman who points out that even among coronary artery patients there are some who are at increased risk for instantaneous death. This group includes those with a left anterior descending coronary artery obstruction and those who have at least a marked two-vessel disease. The conclusion therefore must be that appropriate, *preventive sports medicine studies* should identify the athletes who are at risk and that these athletes should be kept away from the particularly dangerous situations.

This question can be answered reasonably well for the *accident-prone athletic activities*, since careful statistics for these are kept and eventually all deaths are reported that occur during those particular activities. The situation is very much more problematic in the so-called "incidental deaths," since in these there is frequently no autopsy, since not all deaths are reported, and since there are usually no statistics as to how many athletes of a given age or a given high-risk group participate in any one athletic activity. As far as the data are concerned about the particular forms of athletics that certain authors consider to be particularly beneficial or particularly dangerous for the heart, we find mostly arbitrary and dogmatic statements.

For instance, Keren (1981) states that: "Sudden death is more frequent in certain types of sports, notably in those, which require a prolonged tolerance as in marathon runs." On the other hand, the long-distance run is defended, frequently on nothing better than ideologic grounds.

Munschek (1975) and Jung (1982) emphasize that none of the deaths in their series occurred among long-distance runners. Such statements sometimes belong in a pseudoreligious realm. They can be found in the pronouncements of the "jogging-masses" in the American literature, as for instance when Bassler (1972) states that: "No active marathon runner has ever died of a myocardial infarct." This author claims that marathon running "immunizes" against arteriosclerosis.

Such statements are obviously wide of the mark. It is precisely the large number of joggers in the United States that swells the number of reports about sudden deaths during running. Waller (1980) described the findings in five men, aged 40 to 53, who ran regularly between 22 and 176 km/week and who died while running. None of these had a history of coronary artery disease at the time they started running. Autopsy showed far advanced coronary heart disease. Green (1976) described a marathon runner who during the Boston marathon suffered a severe infarct and subsequently died. The autopsy confirmed the extensive infarction, without, however, showing any significant arteriosclerotic changes in the coronary vessels.

Yet, such sudden deaths are rare in running. The statistics assembled by Jung (1982) analyzing 86 so-called "incidental" deaths during a 5-year period in Nordrhein-Westfalen show that only one man died during a running meet, but 43 men died during soccer. However, as already emphasized earlier, since it is not known how many men in the high-risk groups run or play soccer, which is the favorite athletic activity in the German Federal Republic, such statistical data are inadequate to draw any far-reaching conclusions. For instance, Vuori (1978) reports 67 sudden deaths during sauna. This is certainly less of an indication of the dangers of sauna than of the popularity of this activity among Finns.

Other forms of athletics are also frequently denounced as being particularly dangerous to the circulation. These include all those that require sudden and vigorous sprints, and those which require a sudden, severe muscular effort. There is, however, no epidemiologic evidence that these forms of athletics are dangerous to the heart. Even the frequently voiced opinion that deaths during sports are always due to unaccustomed and very high stresses cannot be supported from the literature. The cases described by Waller (1980) are limited to athletes who were well trained and accustomed to the distances which they ran. Friedman (1973) also emphasized the fact that the deaths described by him usually occurred during moderate exercises that were well within the ability of the affected persons.

The goal in trying to prevent sudden deaths in athletics should therefore not be directed toward generalized recommendations about certain forms of athletics or toward "reasonable stress," but toward identifying the particularly *high-risk participants*. In this regard the statistics are reasonably consistent. The sudden death in athletics is predominantly the "prerogative" of the elderly male. Among the 111 deaths due to organic pathology described by Jung (1982), there were only two women, even though women constitute 25% of the membership of the athletic associations. Jung finds the highest incidence of deaths due to organic pathology (28%) in the fifth decade of life. If one considers that this age group is relatively rarely very active in athletics, this further emphasizes the high-risk status of the group. In Vuori's series of deaths during skiing, only one was under 40 years of age (1978). The studies of Vuori further show that in over 90% of the cases in the group over 40 years of age, the cause of sudden death was coronary artery disease.

These data lead to the conclusion

that preventive sports medicine should be directed toward the prevention of sudden cardiac death and particularly toward the man older than 40 years of age. In this person, the principal attention must be directed toward the early detection of coronary artery disease. In addition to routine clinical examination, this person should also have a stress test. It is well known that the resting electrocardiogram (ECG) may be normal in more than half of the persons with a documented single coronary artery narrowing of 50% (Ascoop, 1971). The accuracy of diagnosis can be significantly improved with an *exercise ECG*. With careful selection of the high-risk groups, an *exercise ECG* will demonstrate coronary perfusion disturbances with a reliability of 90%. The exercise ECG is also very suitable for the discovery of dangerous, stress-induced arrhythmias, which, as discussed above, are primarily responsible for the instantaneous cardiac deaths during ath-

letic activity. For these reasons, an exercise ECG should be a mandatory part of any prophylactic sports medicine examination in the older male who wishes to be active in sports. The age limit should be 40 years, although consideration may be given to males over 30. The surprising results of such a prophylactic athletic health examination are given in Figure 4–1. For the best way to perform a stress test exam, the reader is referred to an earlier, comprehensive review (Rost and Hollman, 1982).

Besides prophylactic testing, the high-risk groups should be under *medical supervision during athletic activity*. This is particularly true for the coronary group. The questionnaire of Haskell (1982) shows that such medical presence can significantly reduce the number of cardiac deaths occurring during athletic training sessions with coronary patients in the U.S. During 1.63 million so-called athletic patient hours, there were 50

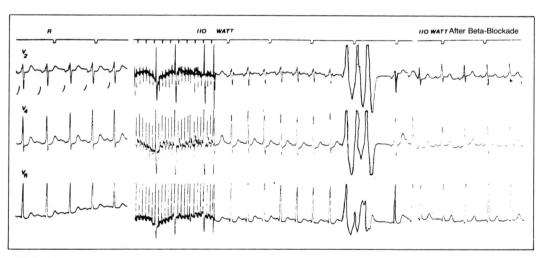

FIG 4–1.

An electrocardiogram (ECG) example to support the need for prophylactic sports-medicine assessment. This ECG was obtained in such a study from a 45-year-old apparently healthy and symptom-free male athlete. The resting ECG *(left)* shows no abnormality. Under 110-watt load *(middle)*, ventricular premature beats become evident even on slow paper speed. On a faster paper speed tracing, runs of ventricular

premature beats become obvious, which forced the immediate discontinuation of the study. On a repeat study after the administration of a beta-blocker, no arrhythmia was observed *(right)*. This tracing also shows that the repolarization disturbance that could be seen during the stress test on lead V_6 had disappeared.

cases of cardiac arrest of which, thanks to immediate medical intervention, 42 were successfully resuscitated.

The picture of *cardiac risks in the young athlete* is considerably more fuzzy, but even here coronary artery disease appears as a primary cause of death. In the series of Munschek (1977) 16 of 39 athletes who died during athletic activity before their 30th birthday had coronary artery disease as the primary cause of death. The other important causes of death were myocarditis in six cases; cardiac anomalies, e.g., anomalous vessels, three cases; and aortic stenosis in only one case, even though this last one is frequently considered to be a major risk factor. In three cases a virus infection and/or tonsillitis was found and was held responsible for a fatal, toxic, cardiovascular collapse. In a separate, second study, Munschek again emphasizes the importance of *myocarditis* as a cause of death in the young athlete. He describes 10 cases of sudden deaths in athletes between the ages of 16 and 35 who died during physical activity because of an inflammatory heart condition.

In this context it is interesting to note that the spectrum of the causes of deaths in the young athlete is changing. These changes are not really changes in the spectrum of disease but lie more in the area of pathologic emphasis and pathologic knowledge concerning the cardiomyopathies. It is surprising that the studies of Munschek (1977) do not show a single case of hypertrophic cardiomyopathy, a condition that was heavily emphasized by Maron (1980). The widely discussed findings of Maron proved first of all that the heart played a most important role in the sudden death of young athletes. There was only one single case, in a series of 29 young athletes, who died suddenly, in which no cardiac pathology was found. Twenty-two of these young athletes actually died during vigorous physical exercise. In 22 of the 29 cases,

death was clearly due to cardiac causes, and in six this seemed very likely. Among the cases that were clearly attributable to cardiac causes, 14, i.e., every other one, could be explained on the basis of cardiac myopathy. Even though there were some clinical indications, the diagnosis was made only rarely prior to the cardiac death. Among the wrong diagnoses, the designation of "athlete's heart" appears in some instances.

Among the dubious cardiac changes, which could not be clearly identified as a sufficient cause of death, there was one case of hypoplastic coronary arteries and five cases of idiopathic, left ventricular, concentric hypertrophy, which could not be definitely classified as an athletic cardiac hypertrophy. The other causes of death were listed as: arteriosclerotic heart disease, 3; aortic ruptures, 2; and two anomalous left coronary arteries. It is interesting that the classic lesions of aortic stenosis and myocarditis do not appear in this series. It must remain an open question as to whether the differences in Munschek's series and Maron's series are due to a difference in the groups studied (Munschek studied primarily average-caliber athletes, while Maron studied high-performance, championship-caliber athletes), or to a fundamental difference in the pathologic evaluation of the findings. In any case, the findings of Maron in the young athletes should focus our attention on the hypertrophic cardiomyopathy. In this context, reference is made to the section on "Echocardiographic Findings."

After discussing the possibility of cardiac deaths during athletic activity, on the basis of preexisting pathology, the question must be asked if whether or not heavy physical stress can damage the healthy heart to the extent of leading to cardiac arrest or to irreversible cardiac damage such as myocardial infarction. On this point, the general opinion is summarized by Aigner (1981): "The determination, that the healthy and well trained heart cannot be damaged by athletic stress is correct, beyond any doubt." This opinion is based primarily on the findings of Jokl (1971) who in the first major study on the etiology of death in athletes reached the conclusion quoted in the heading of this chapter, namely, that the autopsy in athletes who died suddenly always revealed some pathologic cause.

This opinion, however, is certainly not without some serious doubt. Aigner, who strongly supported this point of view, reported a case in the same publication of a long-distance runner who 2 days after having run the marathon, collapsed and died, and in whom the autopsy revealed no apparent cause of death. Among the 35 athletes described by Kirch (1935, 1936), there were three who died suddenly. Two died at rest, one during exercise, and in none of them was a sufficient cause found at autopsy. Reference has already been made to the statistics of Moritz (1946) that included a number of young soldiers who died suddenly, frequently under considerable physical stress, and who failed to reveal any organic pathology.

In some of these deaths, there must have been some *additional etiologic factors* that could cause death, even in healthy persons, and that have to be considered as physical damage, very similar to physical trauma. Mention is made in the literature of such things as cold, heat, drugs (doping), and the combination of altitude hypoxia and physical exercise. *Heat exhaustion* is mentioned prominently in this connection. Under the heading of *drugs*, particular reference is made to the stimulants, which tend to eliminate the natural limits set by fatigue and thus lead to an exhaustion of the protection provided by the so-called *autonomic reserves*. This can lead to total exhaustion and to the failure of the cardiac musculature. The decreased partial pressure of oxygen at high altitudes can lead

to a relative coronary insufficiency even in a normal coronary system when under severe cardiac stress. Kuramoto (1967) reported the appearance of ST segment depression in athletes in Mexico City. Lollgen (1973) published the case of an oarsman who suffered a myocardial infarction when training at high altitude, even though he had a normal coronary artery system.

The next question is whether or not physical stress is sufficient to trigger a myocardial infarction at low altitude. This suggestion seems to be substantiated by such cases as the one reported by Green, in which a runner, with unremarkable coronary arteries, suffered a fatal cardiac infarction. In an attempt to find an explanation for this finding, Samek (1982) analyzed the findings in a group of young patients who had infarctions in the absence of coronary artery disease. He found that in those who died under physical stress there was evidence of *a change in the normal coagulation mechanism*. In some cases in which the autopsy failed to reveal a sufficient cause of death, more careful investigations may well have discovered a more convincing explanation. Thus, James (1967) found in two dead athletes that it took very special histopathologic studies to reveal the presence of some changes in the arterial supply to the sinus node, which was held responsible for the sudden death. Morales described an *intramural* left anterior descending coronary artery, inadequately perfused, when the heart muscles were contracting very vigorously under heavy physical stress condition, as a possible cause of death. In other cases we must assume the presence of arrhythmias, which can occasionally be seen in athletes (see Fig 3–28), and that can lead to ventricular fibrillation in the presence of electrolyte shifts. In the final analysis, the question of whether sudden cardiac arrest can occur in the healthy young athlete, or whether there has to be some underlying pathology, is a philosophical one. According to the principle of causality, there has to be a reason why the healthy heart that is normally capable of adapting to extreme loads fails in an infinitesimally small number of cases under similar circumstances. These cases are so rare that, according to the findings of Moritz (1946), their occurrence during physical exercise may be a purely coincidental one. On the other hand, the discussion presented earlier of the possible pathogenetic mechanisms clearly suggests that in every tragic death of a young athlete, there has to remain a strong suspicion of some underlying etiologic explanation. In view of the rarity of these cases, and the very large number of athletes, such incidents will never be entirely avoidable, even with the most careful preventive measures.

On the other hand, *prophylactic physical examinations* should be performed most carefully and in relation to the degree of anticipated stress. They should therefore be performed with quite particular care in the high-performance athlete. Any suspicion of even a trivial cardiac involvement, e.g., an inflammatory process in connection with tonsillitis, should be taken much more seriously in an athlete than in the general population.

Finally, we must answer the question posed at the beginning of this chapter, namely, whether the cardiac changes, hypertrophy, and increased vagal tone caused by physical conditioning are sufficient by themselves to produce increased risks to the heart. In this connection we must refer to the section on "Historic Overview and Evaluation" of the athlete's heart, since this condition has always been a subject of deep suspicion by virtue of its manifold deviations from the norm. These suspicions can be well illustrated by a quotation from Keren (1981), which is particularly pertinent in this context:

Sudden death affects both active and inactive populations though it appears to be more frequent among sportsmen. This seems to be due to the changes which constitute the so called "athlete's heart," and occur as a result of physical exercise, namely, hypertrophy of the left heart, bradycardia, disturbances of the intraventricular conduction, and, in some cases Wolff-Parkinson-White syndrome. Extreme bradycardia may cause a lengthening of the QT segment of the ECG, as well as electrical instability, thus leading to arrhythmias.

Such a thesis lacks all epidemiologic foundations. Among the deaths occurring in connection with athletics in Nordrhein-Westfalen during a 5-year period, as reported by Jung (1982), there was not one single such case in a high-performance athlete. The relative number of cardiac deaths may well be lower in high-performance athletes than in the average, physically active person. This may be due to the much more thorough medical surveillance in the former group. In the section on "Electrocardiographic Findings" I have made reference to the fact that contrary to the popular belief, the incidence of arrhythmias, even by Holter monitoring, was rarer in our studies in the athlete, in spite of increased vagal tone, than in the nontrained person.

THE TRAUMATIC CARDIAC INJURIES

The last point that must be discussed in the context of potential athletic cardiac injuries is *cardiac trauma*, i.e., contusion of the heart and traumatic myocardial infarction. Exact figures concerning the incidence of such events are not available. Deaths due to cardiac trauma are rare. None appear in the statistics of Munschek or of numerous other authors. In the studies of Jung (1982), nevertheless, there were three cases of deaths due to cardiac contusion in Nordrhein-Westfalen during a 5-year period.

According to the literature, cardiac injuries that are due to athletic events represent only a small percentage of the traumatic myocardial infarctions. The large majority of the reported cases are the result of traffic accidents. Yet, relatively minor injuries in athletics can undoubtedly trigger a myocardial infarction. The fact that young and previously apparently healthy athletes can suffer a traumatic cardiac infarction becomes an important issue in any discussion about the prerequisite for an existing arteriosclerotic condition. In these discussions, it was very much doubted whether or not such a traumatic infarction was even possible in the absence of such a preexisting arteriosclerotic condition. We observed the case of a goalkeeper of a soccer team in the first professional league who, after a collision with an opposing forward, suffered an infarct, which then led to the development of an apical aneurysm. Angiography revealed unremarkable coronary arteries. This case, and similar cases described in the literature, make it obvious that the requirement of preexisting coronary artery disease is not tenable.

In discussing the *pathogenesis of traumatic infarctions,* it is still an open question whether or not these are the result of a primary vascular injury or of a direct myocardial injury, or whether both mechanisms are responsible. Reports concerning direct injury of the coronary arteries usually refer to the descending branch of the left coronary artery. It is assumed that the mechanism of injury involves arterial tears, intimal tears with thromboses, arterial spasm, and subintimal hemorrhage; the latter most commonly under atheromatous plaques. In any case, a preexisting arteriosclerosis is strongly favored. In this connection, *expert opinion* is divided between those who favor arteriosclerosis versus direct trauma in such athletic injuries, particularly in the older athlete. In the individual instances the temporal relationship must be considered (Zimmermann, 1978).

The formerly more prevalent terms *commotio* or *contusio cordis* assume the existence of direct cardiac trauma. By analogy with cerebral injuries, "commotio" refers to reversible lesions and "contusio" refers to irreversible damage, characterized by elevated enzymes and ECG changes. The discussion concerning the pathogenetic mechanism cannot be decided in favor of a myocardial etiology purely by finding normal coronary arteries on arteriography, since a coronary artery thrombus may well have been dissolved by the time the angiography was performed.

Concerning the causation of traumatic infarctions during athletic activities, blunt, external trauma is usually held responsible. This occurs most commonly in the so-called contact sports. The popularity of soccer in Germany explains why most of these injuries occur in goalkeepers, as did the case described above. Other authors described similar cases (De Feyter, 1977; O'Neill, 1981). The anxiety felt by the goalkeeper at the time of an 11 meter penalty kick is well justified for this very reason. Besides direct trauma, indirect pressure injuries of the heart are also possible. Reindell (1960) observed cardiac injuries in wrestlers, which were caused by excessively forceful holds and consequent sharp increases in intrathoracic pressure. In this context, those infarcts that occurred during *weight lifting* were also classsified as being due to mechanical injury (Fox, 1980). Whether this is indeed so must remain an open question and it is debatable whether hemodynamic changes occasioned by the Valsalva maneuver may not be more contributory to the myocardial infarction than the direct effects of raised intrathoracic pressure. For the hemodynamic changes caused by the Valsalva maneuver, see the section entitled "The Valsalva Maneuver."

From a clinical point of view, it should be noted that according to our experience, infarctions caused by athletic activity are frequently missed. In athletes who collapse after blunt thoracic trauma, the possibility of cardiac injury is frequently ignored and no ECG tracing is obtained. If later studies show ECG changes, these are usually not causally connected to the earlier blunt trauma. It is apparent from a review of the literature that traumatic cardiac injuries frequently lead to the development of *aneurysms*, as they did in the case described above. The clinical course of these injuries is frequently characterized by the appearance of all sorts of arrhythmias and conduction defects.

5

Athletics and the Cardiac Patient

With respect to the treatment of this complaint I have little or nothing to advance . . . I knew one who set himself a task of sawing wood, for half an hour every day, and was nearly cured.

Heberden, 1772

The great frequency of cardiovascular disease—every other German dies of it—and the great popularity of athletics—every other German participates in them—necessarily raises the question as to what extent cardiac patients can engage in athletics. Even before this question could be properly examined, the view has prevailed that under certain conditions cardiac patients not only can participate in athletics, but should as a beneficial part of therapy. This is particularly pertinent for the patient with coronary artery disease and for those who have survived a myocardial infarction. While there is considerable experience with these two conditions, there are practically no data concerning the desirability of patients with other forms of heart disease participating regularly in athletic activities. The other heart conditions are myocarditis, cardiomyopathies, congenital defects, and acquired valvular disease. The importance of athletics in rehabilitation is also markedly increasing for those patients whose condition is amenable to surgical correction. These include valvular procedures, aneurysm resections, pacemaker insertions, etc. In these conditions the problem of physical exercise is quite different than in coronary artery disease, and only theoretical advice can be given, since there is not enough practical experience available at this time.

The common denominator for athletic activity in the cardiac patient and for athletic activity in the healthy person is whatever justification there is for athletic activity in general. Athletics is an important factor in improving the quality of life. The question whether athletics is "healthy" is difficult to answer, since it is difficult to define *"health."* Health certainly means more than being "not sick." An expanded concept of health must include the ability to fully realize the human potential, even in the area of physical activity. The aim to improve physical fitness is a legitimate endeavour for the cardiac patient, provided that it does not cause further damage to the heart. The justification of athletic activity in the cardiac patients lies only partly in *improving physical fitness*, but more particularly, in reestablishing the physical fitness that was lost during extended bed-rest, surgical procedures, etc., as part of the general framework of the rehabilitation program.

In this context, physical fitness applies not only to the performance of the heart, but to the performance of the body as a whole. Precisely those activities that are not related to cardiac fitness, such as mobility, coordination, and speed, can be improved by athletic exercise. As far as cardiac performance is concerned, in the past, the engineering principle was applied that stated that the damaged part of a machine had to be treated with the greatest of care. In machines, continued usefulness can only be assured by decreasing utilization. In the biological system different principles must be applied. Muscle, including cardiac muscle, must have a certain functional stress, in order to perform to its best ability. For this reason, even the sick heart needs an adequate functional stimulus, which should, however, never be so great as to be harmful.

In justifying athletic activity for the cardiac patient, reference must be made to the very important *psychic benefits* that can be achieved. It is well known that in cardiac patients the concern about their heart frequently outweighs the significance of the cardiac lesion itself. The realization that they still possess a considerable potential for performance helps these patients to overcome their self-image as a "cardiac cripple."

PHYSICAL CONDITIONING AS A PROPHYLAXIS AGAINST CARDIAC DISEASE

Before discussing the basic theme of this chapter, namely athletics and the cardiac patient, it is desirable to discuss briefly the possibility of preventing such cardiac illness by regular physical activity. A comparatively brief discussion of this matter is made desirable by the enormous literature on the subject, which cannot, and should not, be reviewed at this time. The interested reader is referred to a review written by our group (Hollmann, 1983).

The question concerning the value of athletics in promoting good health, touched on in this section, is largely a philosophical rather than a medical one. It is usually answered on the basis of individual perspective and of sociocultural background, rather than on the basis of facts. While in public discussions it is axiomatic today that athletics have a beneficial effect on health, but it was held with equal conviction in the 19th century that high-performance athletic activity must lead to a premature deterioration of the circulation. This was discussed in detail in connection with the athlete's heart in the section on "Historical Overview and Evaluation." At a time when physical work was a part of earning a living, and was considered to be similar to pain and suffering, such an attitude was just as natural as its opposite is today. In our society there are only a few occupations that require significant bodily work; this is now carried over into the leisure hours. The ability to engage in athletics is therefore viewed as desirable, and for this reason, perhaps also "good" for health.

This general discussion about the usefulness of athletics in promoting health is focused particularly on the possibility of *preventing myocardial infarction* through physical activity. This trend is symbolized by the current slogans of "long distance runners live longer" and "run away from your infarct." This development becomes understandable when we consider the increasing incidence of cardiocirculatory disease in the mortality statistics of the German Federal Republic and of many of the other industrialized nations. The cardiocirculatory diseases represent more than 50% of the death rate and the incidence of deaths due to infarctions has risen disproportionately. Every third cardiocirculatory death and every sixth overall death is due to coronary artery disease. Since this development is quite evidently the result of our form of civilization, it seems natural to blame our physical inactivity as a major contributor.

Although there are numerous indications for the accuracy of this theory through experimental and epidemiologic studies, it must be stated that so far there is no definite proof that one can "run away" from a myocardial infarction. The major difficulty in finding such proof lies in the fact that arteriosclerosis has a very complex etiology that has not yet been fully elucidated. There are apparently a large number of mutually interacting etiologic factors among which the importance of inactivity has not yet been established with any precision.

The difficulty of obtaining such proof becomes particularly clear from *epidemiologic studies*. In these little distinction is usually made between the different forms of physical activity, such as occupational activity or the various athletic endeavours. Furthermore, there is to date no study that is free of the serious question of sampling bias. The question still remains of whether to deal with a problem of selection or a problem of prevention. As long as this question remains unanswered, the effects of athletics on health will remain an open question. To put it in other words: are athletes healthy because they engage in athletics or do athletes engage in athletics because they are healthy?

These problems appear already in the first, and perhaps, classic epidemiologic study by Morris (1953). His studies on the employees of the London public transportation system revealed that the drivers had a much higher incidence of coronary artery disease than the conductors. It appeared to be a logical conclusion that the conductors who had to climb the steep steps of the double-decker buses many times each day were protected by this physical activity from myocardial infarction. Later studies contradicted this view and revealed that the drivers demonstrated significantly increased risk factors already at the time of employment, and may well have self-selected for a less strenuous occupation.

Without going into the details of the numerous studies that are performed in this area, it can be stated that even the most recent ones summarized by Heyden (1981) fail to come to any conclusion regarding the problem of selection. As an example I wish to mention the particularly well-known study by Paffenbarger (1979) using longshoremen as the study group. This study shows that the risk of infarction is inversely proportional to the energy expenditure per week, related to physical labor. The minimal incidence of infarct was found when 2,000 to 3,000 kcal/week were spent in physical work. But even here the question must remain open as to whether or not longshoremen represent an unusually healthy group and whether or not those who develop any signs or symptoms of cardiac disease rapidly abandon this highly strenuous activity. In addition, there are other studies that failed to show such a positive effect of physical activity, such as the epidemiologic study of Hickey (1975), performed in Ireland.

Even though there are still doubts on this subject from a strictly scientific point of view, the available data from the epidemiologic studies are sufficiently convincing to justify the assumption that physical training is an important factor in preventing myocardial infarction. This is particularly true if training is not taken in isolation but as a part of a general, health-conscious, rational lifestyle. It caused a considerable and justifiable stir when it was found from the mortality statistics that coronary artery deaths were on the decline in the United States, con trary to the experience of the European industrialized nations. Even though one could counter with the observation that the relative number of coronary artery deaths is still higher in the United States than in Western Europe, the decreasing incidence does show that the adoption of a health-conscious lifestyle can reverse the frightening rise in cardiocirculatory mortality.

The causes for this positive development in the United States are of a complex nature and cannot be attributed solely to the ever-increasing number of joggers as the long-distance runners would like us to believe. Additional, and very important, reasons include changes in the dietary patterns of the average American, away from the ingestion of large amounts of animal fats and carbohydrates (Heyden, 1981), a decrease in the per capita consumption of cigarettes, and a better compliance of the American population with the sound pharmacologic management of hypertension. Possibly one of the reasons for this *increased health consciousness* of the American public can be found in the poor national health insurance system in that country. The perfect health insurance system in the German Federal Republic causes the individual to take a somewhat cavalier attitude toward his own health. The average citizen gives little thought to sickness prevention or health maintenance, and believes that having made his contribution to the Health Insurance Fund, he has done all that is necessary. If he then has the first indications of a coronary artery problem, or even of an infarct, it comes as a great surprise to him that there is no ready remedy for his problem.

The value of physical conditioning in the prevention of the infarct epidemic must be appraised in two ways. It may well have direct benefits, but, more probably, its benefits are indirect and act by making larger segments of the population conscious of, and interested in, improving their health. One can assume that anyone who is disciplined enough to run, bicycle, or swim regularly also has a positive attitude toward his health, keeps his weight down, and limits his use of cigarettes. Besides epidemiologic data, and general reflections on the value of physical activity, sports medicine has also gathered a number of *experimental data* during the last few decades that indicate that a sensible amount of athletic activity is obviously a reasonable thing to do. Even though it is an open question of whether or not athletics have a direct preventive role against cardiac infarction, it can be assumed that a circulatory system develops increased reserves through endurance training, and is thus in a better position to withstand the onset of cardiac disease. The so-called HIP (heart insurance plan) study showed that those of the insured population who were physically active still suffered myocardial infarcts, but that the incidence of sudden deaths or of fatal infarcts was significantly less than in the physically inactive group (Shapiro, 1965). Physical activity also has additional beneficial effects on other risk factors, particularly on obesity, diabetes mellitus, and hypertension, through increased calorie utilization.

A particularly interesting approach in recent years was found in the study of *fat metabolism.* For a long time, the discussions were limited to a consideration of whether or not athletic activity could lower the cholesterol levels. In the meantime, it was found that it raised the *HDL-cholesterol* levels, i.e., that fraction of the total cholesterol that was believed to be protective against arteriosclerosis. Another important experimental finding that must be emphasized is the *increase in fibrinolysis* under the influence of physical exercise. If one assumes that thrombus formation has an important role in the pathogenesis of infarction, then this observation may well be significant from a prophylactic point of view (for a review of the literature, see Hollmann, 1983).

In summary, the question of whether

or not it is possible to run away from a myocardial infarct must be answered by saying that to some extent there are very strong arguments for it. On the other hand, the thesis that long-distance runners live longer has never been proved. Longevity appears to be more a function of genetic composition, than of physical activity. It is possible that the effects of physical activity are only indirect in nature and that the same results could be obtained by leading a sensible life and eating a sensible diet. For this reason, there appears to be no necessity to make athletics an obligatory and dogmatic part of a healthy way of life for those patients who belong to a vigorous *anti-athletic group*. This latter group can find consolation in the words of Churchill, who, when asked the secret of his longevity, answered: "No sports, only whisky."

If a healthy person wishes to use athletic activity as a preventive against an infarct, the physician should not just recommend participation in athletics, but should give specific recommendations, the most important of which are summarized below.

Engaging in athletics for the sake of health assumes that this activity will not be detrimental to health. This means that there has to be a careful *prior physical assessment* from a *sports medicine point of view*. This is even more important if there is a possibility of a preexisting illness. For this reason, before any older person, and particularly any man over 40 years of age, engages in athletic activity, he or she must be carefully examined, including a stress electrocardiogram (ECG). These studies must be repeated at regular intervals, as long as the person continues to participate in athletics. As explained in the section on "Nontraumatic Cardiac Injuries," the most frequent cause of sudden death in athletics was coronary artery disease that may not be discovered during "at rest" examinations.

If there are no health-related objections to starting conditioning, considera-

tion has to be given to the *optimal form, intensity, and duration* of the exercise. In considering the exercise that is optimal for the cardiocirculatory system, there are many misconceptions. As described in the section on "The Function of the Athlete's Heart," only *endurance exercise* will have an effect on the cardiocirculatory system. To achieve any effect this stress must reach a certain minimal intensity, frequency, and duration.

The desirable *minimal intensity* is given by the so-called *exercise pulse frequency* of 180 minus age. This means that a 50-year-old should reach a pulse frequency of 130 beats per minute under stress in order to achieve any beneficial results from the conditioning. *Walking or gardening* are forms of "stress" that are frequently, but mistakenly, considered to be beneficial for the circulation. Concerning the desirable *minimal time*, the studies in the Cologne Institute for Circulation Research and Sports-medicine have shown that the stimulus had to be maintained for at least 5 minutes, and preferably 10 minutes to become effective on the circulation (Hollmann, 1983).

The more recent aspects of the relationship of physical activity and metabolism have shown that the minimal exercise time had to be further extended for physical activity to be fully useful. The results obtained in the study of Paffenbarger show clearly that the optimal preventive effects of athletics are realized only if physical activity uses up at least 300 to 400 kcal per day. This would correspond to a cross-country run of 30 to 40 minutes, in the absence of any other physical activity.

On the other hand, this study also shows that further increases in physical activity do not increase its prophylactic benefits. The occasionally encountered statement that "the one who runs the longest distances is the best protected against myocardial infarction" is certainly not true. Running 100 to 200 km per week increases performance but does not increase longevity. Contrary to the beliefs of some long-distance running enthusiasts, a rational moderation must be sought in this form of physical activity as well.

The table in Figure 5–1 contains concrete recommendations concerning the speed of running. If a 50-year-old reaches the training pulse frequency at 150 watts, this means a run of 150 m/minute and a time of 6½ minutes for 1000 m, assuming that his weight is 70 kg. If the person is heavier, i.e., requires a greater energy output for the same running speed, the duration of the run must be correspondingly lengthened. In order to avoid mis-

WATT \ kg	50	60	70	80	90	100
75	8	9	10	–	–	–
100	7	8	9	10	–	–
125	6	7	8	9	10	–
150	5	6	7	8	8,5	9
175	4,5	5,5	6	7	7,5	8
200	4	4,5	5	6	6,5	7

Established Exercise Groups

WATT \ kg	50	55	60	65	70	75	80	85	90	95	100	105	110	115
50	95	90	85	80	75	70	70							
60	105	100	90	85	80	75	75	70						
70	115	110	100	95	90	85	80	75	75	70				
80	125	115	110	100	100	90	85	80	75	75	70	70		
90	135	125	115	110	105	95	90	90	85	80	75	75	70	70
100	145	135	125	120	110	105	100	95	90	85	80	80	75	75
110	155	145	135	125	115	110	105	100	95	90	85	85	80	75
120	165	155	140	135	125	120	110	105	100	95	90	90	85	80
130	175	165	150	140	130	125	120	110	105	110	95	95	90	85
140	190	175	160	150	140	135	125	120	115	110	105	100	95	95
150	200	185	170	160	150	140	130	125	120	115	110	105	100	95

Exercise groups (left margin, top to bottom): 3, 2, 1
Exercise Groups Determined by Nomogram (bottom): 1, 2, 3, 4

FIG 5–1.
Table to convert the bicycle ergometric performance into running speeds (after Lagestroem, 1975). The upper part of the table shows the running speeds as the time required to run 1,000 m. This is particularly appropriate for the mass athlete. A subject weighing 60 kg who can reach a 150-watt load at the ideal pulse rate of 180 minus age in years should accomplish 1000 meters in 6 minutes. At a weight of 70 kg, because of the larger mass that has to be moved, the 1,000 meters should take 7 minutes. In the lower part the same table is shown, but the speed of running is given in m/minute. This is particularly useful in cardiac rehabilitation.

understandings, it must be mentioned that the training pulse rate of 180 minus age is just a minimal guide line for the nontrained person. The trained person, by virtue of his improved metabolic adaptation, should be exposed to a higher percentage of his maximal exercise potential in order to gain further benefits from the exercise. Thus, championship-caliber athletes can maintain physical activity at 180 to 200 pulse rates for 1 to 2 hours. As far as the *frequency of the exercise* is concerned, it should be noted that a biologic stimulus is more effective if more often applied. Running 10 minutes each day is more effective than running for 70 minutes on the weekend. Exercise-physiologic studies have shown that the minimal effective frequency should be at least three times per week.

FUNCTIONAL CARDIOCIRCULATORY DISEASE

The Hyperkinetic Heart Syndrome, Dyscardia, and Hypotension

Functional disturbances of the cardiocirculatory system are the most frequent diagnoses in the practice of cardiology. It is precisely in this group that drug therapy is far less effective than a carefully planned psychologic and physical therapy program, in which physical exercise takes a place of pride. These diagnoses include functional disturbances that, depending on the point of view of the observer, were classified as primarily psychologic or primarily functional. They were labeled hyperkinetic heart syndrome, dyscardia, cardiophobia, etc. It is in these patients, who, from an irrational fear of a myocardial infarction, have practically immobilized themselves that the experience of surviving graded physical exercise with impunity, is particularly beneficial. In primarily psychogenic cardiac syndromes, group athletics should be recommended, i.e., gymnastics or team-play sports, where the fascination of the game overcomes the cardiac symptomatology.

The *hyperkinetic heart syndrome* is characterized by an increased sympathetic drive. In this situation, endurance training is the logical treatment of choice, since this raises the vagal tone and leads to a decrease in the sympathetic tone. It is true, however, that in practice we frequently encounter the problem that these patients commonly develop a severe tachycardia early in exercise, which makes it impossible for them to engage in any long distance running. In this situation the short-term use of a *beta-blocking agent* is indicated that will prevent these excessive tachycardias. This pharmacologic crutch can be discarded as soon as the effects of training become apparent.

The hypotensive complaints represent a group of cardiocirculatory disturbances in which the psychogenic elements predominate over the purely functional ones. There is usually only a very loose connection between *hypotension* and a number of associated complaints. The administration of drugs tends to fixate the patient on his/her self image of "illness," and it is far better to improve circulation through planned activity than to support it with drugs and thus further weaken it.

The hypotensive complaints, and particularly the *orthostatic hypotension*, serve as an excellent example for the illustration of the principle that the thorough understanding of the specific responses of the cardiocirculatory system to the specific effects of the various forms of physical exercise allow a rational, differential utilization of these modalities. The great importance of endurance training has unfortunately led to the idea that only endurance training had beneficial effects on the circulation. While this may be true for the improvement of the range of performance of the cardiocirculatory system, it certainly does not hold for its regulation. It obviously makes no sense to treat the hypotensive patient the same way as the hypertensive patient, and yet, this is done frequently in practice. Such endurance training should, at least in theory, make the hypotensive patient worse.

In these patients, *those exercises* should be used that raise the blood pressure and improve the regulatory mechanics. These include the *"power" athletics, power gymnastics, and team sports,* which all increase blood pressure through tensional stimuli, and those forms of exercise that have a cold temperature stimulus, *like swimming.* In swimming, short distance sprints and diving should be recommended where the cold stimulus is more apparent. Long-distance, endurance swimming should be avoided. In connection with swimming, the heat and cold stimulation of the Finnish sauna must, naturally, be emphasized. From a circulatory physiologic point of view, in this context we must favorably consider certain forms of athletics that are ordinarily not considered to be particularly beneficial. These include *body building, alpine skiing, and riding.* In the last two the danger of injury must be weighed against the positive benefits.

Hypertension

At this point it is appropriate to make at least a brief mention of hypertension, since in its early stages and in its "essential" form, it has to be considered as a functional disturbance. The general, therapeutic measures that are recommended to the hypertensive patient include the initiation of a physical conditioning program, in addition to the traditional weight control, stress-avoidance and, above all, a calm and well-regulated lifestyle. The value placed on such physical conditioning varies widely. Some authors, e.g., Mellerowitz (1974), claim that physical conditioning eliminates the cause of hypertension, at least in its initial phase that is believed to be due to sympathetic hyperactivity. Caution is indicated, however, before accepting such a fundamental role for physical conditioning. Essential hypertension is a disease of unknown etiology and it is inappropriate to consider physical exercise as being directly effective in eliminating the cause of the disease.

For this reason, the effects of training on high blood pressure are viewed variously in the literature. Some authors report positive results (Choquette, 1973; Schwalb, 1974). It must be stated, however, that in most of the available studies, physical conditioning was combined with changes in dietary patterns, rest cures, and drug therapy, so that it is not possible to identify the specific contributions made by any of them. Our own studies showed only a slight decrease in pressure in the young, hypertensive patient and no effect in the older patient (Rost, 1976). It must also be mentioned that contrary to the widely held belief that physical conditioning lowers the hypertension caused by physical exercise, there is no difference in the pressure observed in the trained and the nontrained, given similar stress conditions (Reindell, 1960; Hollmann, 1976).

On the other hand, we frequently see low resting blood pressure values in the trained athlete. The question must then be raised as to whether this can be interpreted as the direct result of training, or whether it is due to the training-induced weight loss. From these thoughts it is apparent that the conclusion can be drawn that training is an important adjuvant in the management of hypertension, even though a direct blood pressure lowering effect could not be demonstrated to date. As the *mechanism of action of such physical conditioning,* we may consider the reduction in weight, the decrease of sympathetic drive, and the loss of salt through increased perspiration.

We must also add to the general, previously-mentioned reasons, the improved treatment *compliance*, which is particularly important in the hypertensive patient. As is well known, there is hardly any other group of patients with as bad a drug compliance record as the hypertensive patient who has been free of symptoms for some time. It is hoped that regular physical activity will engender a general improvement in the health orientation and behavior of this group.

These considerations do make it clear, however, that physical conditioning cannot replace *drug therapy*. The misconception that the long-distance runner with hypertension no longer needs his medication is unfortunately not borne out in practice. In this connection the question is frequently asked in practice of whether or not the hypertensive patient on drug therapy should continue athletic activity and whether or not any particular drug therapy should be preferred. This question will be discussed in the section on "Physical Exercise and Cardiac Drugs." Because of the great importance of this matter, particularly for the hypertensive athlete, a short summary of the prevailing beliefs will be presented at this time. The possibility of engaging in athletics while on drug therapy depends, in the individual case, on the severity of the hypertensive disease, on the medication being used, and on the intensity of the athletic activity. In the *hypertensive performance athlete* this question must be answered differently, depending on the form of athletic activity engaged in.

Endurance sports act favorably on hypertension. A moderate hypertension, which does not require drug therapy, is not a contraindication for high-performance endurance sports. Those forms of athletic activity that cause a marked rise in blood pressure, such as *weight lifting* and *rowing* are probably contraindicated. Even though it cannot be proved statistically, the study of champion athletes leaves the impression that in the above-mentioned forms of athletics, the number of hypertensive persons is higher than could be explained by chance. Perhaps these sports do foster the development of hypertension. The same is true for those *team sports* that generate substantial psychic stress, e.g., handball and swimming. If a sports medicine examination reveals the presence of hypertension, the athlete should be advised to abandon the high-performance sport and switch to an endurance sport. Advising a high-performance athlete or oarsman to switch to long-distance running or bicycling is probably not going to be very successful in practice. At least, however, this athlete should be advised to supplement his physical activities with some additional endurance component.

When drug therapy becomes necessary, further participation in high-performance athletics should be forbidden. Today, the high-performance sports require such a high load that perfect health has to be a minimal requirement. When drug therapy is required this condition is no longer met. Only few exceptions can be made and only in those sports that do not require major physical loads (e.g., rifle shooting and dressage riding). The same prohibition applies to drug-dependent endurance athletes, since all antihypertensive medications affect hemodynamics and metabolism.

In severe hypertension, all high-performance athletics are forbidden as a matter of course. The real problems are created by the moderately severe cases. At the present time the β-*blockers* and the *diuretics* are the real problem drugs. To what extent the *calcium channel blockers* will become significant in this regard is not yet known. The side effects of the β-blockers are described in detail in the section on "Physical Exercise and Cardiac Drugs." The most detrimental aspect for the endurance-trained hypertensive athlete is the drug-induced bradycardia that forces him to function constantly at an increased stroke volume. There is a real danger that the resulting cardiac hypertrophy will exceed the normal athlete's heart enlargement. Particularly undesirable are the metabolic side effects, the decrease in fat utilization, and the danger of hypoglycemia. To date, there are no definite experiences as far as the diuretics are concerned. We must assume, however, that the loss of the electrolytes necessary for muscular contraction has undesirable consequences. There is the additional danger that the incidence of arrhythmias is increased by hypokalemia.

The situation is different in leisure-time activities. In this case, if at all justifiable, physical activity should be recommended in addition to drug therapy. The increased vagal tone, due to training, may be synergistic with the β-blocker effects and with the loss of salt through sweating or diuretics. Such training should be recommended only after the hypertension is well controlled with drug therapy. Patients who have a systolic pressure over 180 mm Hg or a diastolic pressure over 120 mm Hg should never be allowed into the field.

In this situation both the resting blood pressure and the pressure under stress must be considered. The *stress pressure* can exceed the resting pressure by a very considerable margin. For the purposes of athletic activity, the results of drug therapy must be tested under ergometric conditions. This was pointed out most effectively by Franz (1979). It also pertains to the choice of the antihypertensive medication. In this context, Franz pointed out that the blood pressure lowering effects of the diuretics were much less under load conditions than those achieved by the β-blockers.

As far as selecting a form of athletics is concerned, the patient with high blood pressure should be guided toward the well-supervised endurance sports. The use of the heart rate as a yardstick is discussed in the section on "Physical Exercise and Cardiac Drugs" and is particularly pertinent for this group of athletes.

CORONARY ARTERY DISEASE

The Postinfarct Patient

Organizational Development

The change in attitude toward the value of physical activity in cardiac patients is best illustrated by the present management of coronary artery disease. While the standard therapy at the time of the great "infarct wave" at the end of the war in the German Federal Republic was rest, as a fundamental principle, today, a sensible and controlled exercise program is widely accepted. In place of the strict bed rest of 6-weeks' duration, which was the rule at the time, we now see *early ambulation*, albeit there are considerable variations on this theme. Ideally, in stable patients, *early and continuous rehabilitation* is provided in a "clinical rehabilitation center." There the resumption of physical exercise is one of the basic therapeutic measures. More and more patients are allowed to participate in increasing physical activity under medical supervision in the so-called *ambulatory coronary artery activity clubs.*

This *rehabilitation sequence* was first introduced in grand style, in the framework of the "Hamburg Model," in the 1970s (Ilker, 1973; Donat, 1974). This model combined the experiences gathered by the first of these groups in the middle 1960s. The first *ambulatory coronary artery activity clubs* were established in the German Federal Republic around 1965 in Schorndorf and Munchen. Under the stimulus of the *Hamburg Model*, which was the first one to show the possibility of using a large athletic club for the benefit of the coronary artery patients, the number of the ambulatory coronary artery activity clubs grew to 80 by 1978. At the time of translating the manuscript for this monograph in 1985, this number has increased to 1,200. This enormous and still growing increase in the development of the ambulatory coronary artery activity groups is good evidence for the ready acceptance of this idea by the patients.

It must be emphasized at this point that this development is fostered primarily by the patients themselves, and that clinical cardiology has still not come to terms with it. The first coronary artery activity club of Schorndorf was established by a physician in the framework of a handicapped persons' athletic club, for which he was providing medical care (Hartmann, 1974). In connection with this development, "based" primarily on the coronary patients themselves, the expression of "voting with one's feet" was most appropriate.

The Advantages

The overwhelming acceptance of this development by the patients is no evidence for its usefulness. In view of the potential risks to which the patient is subjected through physical exercise, and which were discussed in detail in the section on "Nontraumatic Cardiac Injuries," it is not surprising that a number of cardiologists regarded this development with only very moderate enthusiasm. This is particularly true when the physical activities are exaggerated to the point of high-performance athletics. Recommendations, and indeed, promises of complete recovery through running the marathon are unfortunately found not only in the lay press but even in the scientific literature. There are a number of publications in the Anglo-American literature about a series of controlled studies on the marathon run in infarct patients (Bassler, 1972; Dressendorfer, 1979; Kavanagh, 1974).

Such studies prove how well patients can perform after an infarct. They also give an indication that the earlier, extreme immobilization was certainly not always necessary. The true value of these studies, however, is very dubious. There is no evidence for the argument, frequently voiced in favor of such hyperactivity, that only a very high level of training can have a therapeutic effect on arteriosclerosis. The potential danger to such high-risk groups as the postinfarct patients seem to demand that the proof of this thesis be obtained in healthy persons or in patients with less severe manifestations of arteriosclerosis. High-performance athletics are undesirable even on pathophysiologic and sports medical grounds. To produce *cardiac hypertrophy* in postinfarct patients who already have a limited coronary perfusion seems very problematic indeed.

The pronounced potential risk that physical activity carries for the coronary artery patient makes it mandatory to weigh the risk-benefit ratios very carefully. The therapeutic about-face from complete rest to a measured physical exercise must be justified critically and not just by an enthusiasm for athletics. This about-face is not nearly as drastic as it may appear considering the change in attitude against physical exercise that has taken place in the German Federal Republic between the 1950s and today. Heberden, who was the first one to describe coronary artery disease in 1772, already realized the value of physical exercise for his patients with "angina." This is manifest in the quotation at the head of this chapter.

Another pioneer of the motion-therapy was Oertel (1884) who introduced the concept of "terrain therapy." Gotteiner (1968) must be considered another pioneer of the prospective motion-therapy for coronary artery patients in the post-war "infarct-wave," even though the level of activity he required from his patients in Israel would today be considered heroic.

The introduction of exercise therapy

was based on the hope that it may lead to the *development of collateral circulation,* as it has done in some animal experiments (Amann, 1951; Scharper, 1971). Unfortunately the results of animal experiments cannot be transposed to man, and quite particularly not to older men with coronary artery disease. The few longitudinal coronary arteriographic studies, such as those of Conner (1976) or Ferguson (1974) are not encouraging. Their population is small and of questionable validity, since they could not exclude spontaneous vessel development and, furthermore, necessarily contain a built-in sampling error. It is also unlikely that better data will be obtained in the future. Coronary arteriography cannot be justified or even excused on purely scientific grounds, in the context of an athletic training program.

For these reasons, it may be permissible to extrapolate to the coronary artery system arterial perfusion disturbances obtained in the *femoral artery.* An exercise training study, under the direction of Buchwalsky (1974), showed unmistakable clinical improvement, but this could not be explained on the basis of angiographic findings. It seems likely that the improvement in the distances that these patients could walk after physical conditioning was due to a better walking technique and to a metabolic adaptation, which produced less lactic acid under identical load conditions.

There is no *clear evidence* that athletic activity has any beneficial effect on the course of coronary artery disease. Besides there being no evidence for the development of an increased collateral circulation, there is also no evidence that training affects the regression of arteriosclerotic manifestations or that it decreases the reinfarction rate and mortality. The sobering realization of these facts should, hopefully, lead to a decrease in exaggerated expectations and to an equal decrease of exaggerated training. Finally, it should be remembered that this assess-

ment of the value of exercise is parallel to the assessment of drug therapy and surgical therapy. With the exception of β-blockers and coronary artery bypass procedure for left main stem stenosis, there is to date no convincing evidence that drugs or surgery prolong life in these patients.

While there is no evidence that athletic activity affects the course of coronary artery disease, there is no question that it helps the patient to cope with the disease. This is true both in the physical area as well as in the psychologic-social area. The general considerations that led to the recommendation of athletic activity for these patients were discussed in the introduction to this chapter. They are valid for coronary artery patients, even though there is no concrete evidence yet about the effects of this activity on the course of the arteriosclerotic process. The fact that the activity helps the patient to cope with the disease justifies its use, provided that this form of therapy does not endanger the patient.

Beside the *psychic effects* we must point out the improved *economy of the cardiocirculatory system* manifested by a decrease in myocardial oxygen requirements for similar cardiac activity. The mechanisms for this effect were described in detail in the chapter entitled "The Athlete's Heart." The results of our own studies on the hemodynamic effects of training programs in older men is shown in Figure 5–2,A. The sparing effect on circulatory function is shown by the achievement of a similar cardiac output by lower heart rate and increased stroke volume.

It should be pointed out that hemodynamic studies of this type, in healthy volunteers, cannot be applied unconditionally to coronary patients. Controlled hemodynamic studies in coronary patients are, to date, both too few in numbers and also internally contradictory. For example, the studies of Schnellbacher (1972) in coronary artery patients before and after training showed a decrease in *cardiac output* and an increase in *pulmonary artery pressure*, i.e., a deterioration. In contrast, the studies of Ressl (1975) showed that training had no effect on cardiac output and pulmonary artery pressure. Studies performed by Brecht (1981) on our coronary patients showed no effect on pulmonary artery pressure and an insignificant decrease in cardiac output (see Fig 5–2).

The "sparing" of the cardiocirculatory function is best expressed by a reduction of pulse frequency. As discussed in detail in the chapter on "The Athlete's Heart," the reduction in heart rate is a function of peripheral influences, such as the reduction in sympathetic drive through improved muscular metabolism. This can be substantiated in our patients. It seems remarkable that in spite of relatively low training intensity, there is an increasing drop in the lactate levels, indicating a decreased anaerobic energy utilization for identical loads. This was true in studies lasting 2 or more years (Fig 5–3). The groups under our care engage twice each week for 1½ hours in athletic activity, of which only 15 minutes are endurance activity, usually running. This observation substantiates the contention that extensive loads are not necessary to achieve beneficial training effects. The fact that a direct cardiac effect of conditioning, undesirable because of the hypertrophy it causes, is not necessary, can be documented by our studies. We have not observed any cardiac hypertrophy in studies lasting over a period of years (Fig 5–4).

The various arguments concerning the significance of physical conditioning in the context of preventing and rehabilitating coronary artery disease can be found in Table 5–1.

The Disadvantages

In any discussion of the disadvantages, the advantages of supervised exercise therapy in coronary artery patients must be contrasted with the most important and most dramatic *life threatening events*, i.e., the sudden cardiac death and reinfarction occurring during athletic activity. It is statistically proved that the fundamental condition for recommending physical activity to the patients, i.e., the avoidance of increased risks, has been met satisfactorily. As part of the "Hamburg Model" it was shown that the patients who were eligible for the coronary activity clubs and who participated in athletics did not have a higher mortality than those who would have met the admission criteria, but who did not accept an invitation to join the ambulatory coronary activity club. Sanne (1977) found no increase in deaths in the exercising group when compared with the control group. The mortality figures, reported from Hamburg, corresponded with our rate of 1.5% per year, which were derived from the figures of Matschuk (1982) gathered over a period of 6 years. Such a *mortality rate* is clearly under the expected value of 3% to 6%, which was the value predicted for the post infarction group. On the other hand, these figures do not permit the drawing of any conclusions concerning the preventive value of athletics, since the study group is obviously a highly select one.

Even on statistical grounds, *accidents* can be expected to occur during training activities in this high-risk group. In our group, we observed three serious cardiac complications in a 10-year observation period. One death was due to a reinfarction during the exercise period, one was a sudden death in a patient who in addition to the group activity also engaged in solo cross-country running, and one patient who developed ventricular fibrillation during cross-country skiing that could be successfully reversed with repeated defibrillating counter shocks.

Such incidents during athletic activity in coronary patients were also observed and reported by other groups,

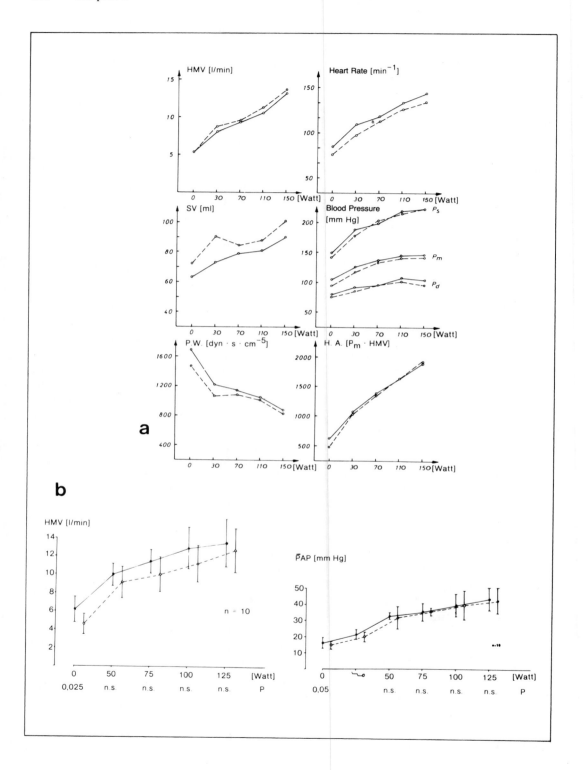

such as Laubinger (1974) from the "Hamburg Model" and also Wieser (1980). In spite of the dramatic effects of the individual incident, the total number of such incidents is surprisingly low, considering the high-risk status of this group. This is substantiated by our experience in Cologne, where it must be mentioned in the context of a quantitative assessment of the described incidents that the number of ambulatory coronary activity clubs has risen to 17, with a regular membership of 300 to 400 patients.

In the section on "Sport Related Risks for the Heart" we have defined the increased risks of sudden death. This incidence can apparently be decreased by careful selection of the patients, and by good medical care of the selected groups. Since physical activity cannot be avoided in daily living, it must be assumed that in the patient in whom the incident occurs in a situation other than athletic activity, it could have just as easily occurred in any other situation. For example, one of our patients who was excluded from further participation in athletics because of a deterioration in his physical condition died suddenly while pushing his car, i.e., a typically high pressure stress. The individually determined and supervised activity within the coronary artery activity clubs, combined with good *medical care*, reduces the risk to a minimum.

On the other hand, the possibility of physical exercise triggering an acute cardiac death can never be entirely eliminated. For this reason it is not only a legal requirement (Rieger, 1979), but a medical requirement as well, that training be provided only in medically supervised and appropriately equipped groups. The need for the presence of a physician, equipped with a *defibrillator,* is demonstrated by reports of successful resuscitations, as indeed in our case described above. The particularly great likelihood of successful resuscitation of ventricular fibrillation occurring during athletic stress is demonstrated in the report of Roskamm (1978). Reporting five such acute incidents during exercise therapy in a rehabilitation center, he was able to resuscitate four patients successfully. We must also again refer to the above mentioned American report by Haskell (1982) who describes 42 successful resuscitations in a series of 50 cardiac arrests. The continuous presence of a well-equipped physician, as recommended in the *Guidelines of the German Association of Sports-physicians* has thus been amply justified in practice (Flothner, 1981).

The second potential detrimental ef-

FIG 5–2.
Studies on the hemodynamic effects of physical conditioning. The first study **(a)** was done on healthy 55- to 70-year-old men. Cardiac output was determined by the dye-dilution technique; blood pressure was measured directly. Physical conditioning was carried out five times each week for a period of 12 weeks. Preconditioning values are shown by the *solid line,* the postconditioning values are indicated by the *broken line.* The results show that at rest and under moderate loads, essentially unchanged cardiac output was accomplished with a lower heart rate and greater stroke volume. The peripheral resistance and mean arterial pressure did not change significantly. **b,** the studies performed by Brecht (1981) on 10 patients in our coronary artery activity group. After a 1- year conditioning period performed twice weekly, there is a nonsignificant decrease in cardiac output under identical load. The mean pulmonary artery pressure rose an average of 40 mm Hg prior to the study. After 1 year of conditioning, this did not change appreciably. The data were obtained by Swan-Ganz catheter. The athletic program included calisthenics, running, and game sports. The studies show that contrary to a number of references in the literature, the cardiac sparing is in the area of rate reduction rather than in the area of cardiac output. The study also shows that carefully prescribed and controlled conditioning does not aggravate a moderately elevated pulmonary artery pressure.

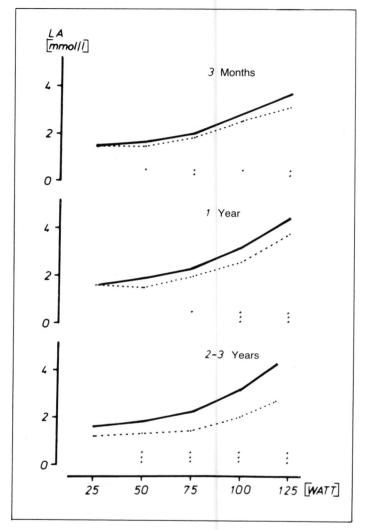

FIG 5–3.

The effect of physical conditioning on the blood lactic acid levels under increasing loads performed in the framework of the ambulatory coronary artery activity club. (Study performed by Matschuk, 1982, in the Cologne coronary artery activity club.) In spite of the brief training periods of only 15 minutes twice weekly, there is an increasing and significant decrease in lactate levels. This becomes more pronounced over a period of 3 months, 1 year, and 2–3 years.

fect to be feared is the development of a *myocardial insufficiency* on the basis of overload during physical conditioning. Roskamm (1978) expressed the fear that in postinfarction patients with a large scar, the remaining myocardium may be overtaxed during physical training. It was observed in a number of individual in-

stances that such patients were driven into myocardial insufficiency. The appearance of infarct-specific changes in more than four ECG leads are considered a *contraindication* for further athletic activity.

In the groups monitored by us, not one case was observed in which athletic

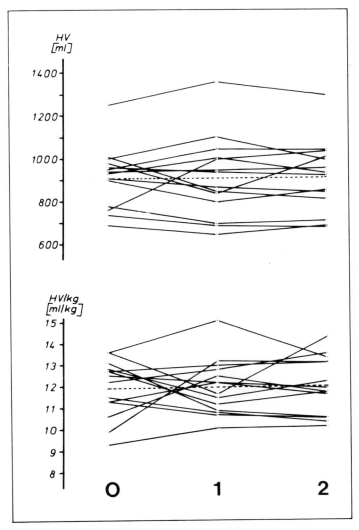

FIG 5–4.
Effect on the absolute and relative cardiac volume in members of the Cologne coronary artery activity club. (Matschuk, 1982.) The control studies were performed after one year *(1)* and over a period of from 2 to 5 years *(2)*. There is no evidence of any significant effect on cardiac volume either in the individual or for the mean value of the group. This was true even in subjects with a distinctly enlarged heart.

activity was responsible for the development of cardiac insufficiency, even in the presence of cardiac enlargement (see Fig 5–4). Obviously such a statement is predicated on a careful selection of the patients and on individually tailored exercise. In cases of excessive load, the appearance of cardiac insufficiency can certainly not be excluded.

In our experience, the resting ECG has very little prognostic value. Even in patients with extensive anterior wall infarcts who met the criteria established by Roskamm (1978), we have not observed any increased complication rates (Matschuk, 1982). In these patients attention must be paid not only to the ECG changes but also to the relatively good individual

TABLE 5–1.

Indications for Athletics in the Prevention and Rehabilitation of Coronary Heart Disease*

Nonmedical indications
   Psychologic factors
   Sociologic factors
   Economic factors
Medical indications
   Improvement of health consciousness (avoidance
     of external risk factors)
   Positive effects on internal risk factors
   Better utilization of performance reserves (better
     coordination)
   Improved capillary and collateral circulation devel-
     opment (?)
   Reduction in the work of the heart
     Pressure
     Volume
     Acceleration
   Decrease of myocardial oxygen utilization

*Summary of the indications for the use of athletics dis-
cussed in the context of prevention or rehabilitation of coronary artery disease. For details, see text.

responses to exercise. Naturally, it is essential in these patients to provide not only very careful monitoring, but also additional diagnostic studies, such as *pulmonary artery pressure measurements*, at rest and under stress.

As a possible negative effect of physical conditioning, Roskamm raised the question of whether too much time was wasted in this activity and patients were kept from indicated and timely surgical repair. In our experience, the opposite is more likely to happen in practice. The intensive involvement of the physician with his patients, particularly during physical activity, allows, in medically well-supervised groups, the early recognition of any deterioration and the prompt referral for coronary angiography.

As a last possible negative effect, the occasional *unfavorable psychologic consequences* must be mentioned. While the favorable psychologic effects are usually emphasized, the unfavorable effects are frequently forgotten. These can arise when a coronary patient observes the deterioration of a fellow member of the group, his reinfarction, or sudden death, either during or independent of athletic activity. Such negative impact can be avoided by appropriate *psychologic counseling*, particularly group discussions.

In weighing these advantages and disadvantages, it must be emphasized that experience, stretching over decades, has clearly shown that athletic activity was an important contribution to the care of the coronary artery patient, in conjunction with other therapeutic maneuvers, and when prescribed in an appropriate form and in an individually tailored fashion. Unfortunately, in practice these cardiologic principles are frequently ignored in the care of these groups. For this reason, the most important selection criteria and the guidelines for the practical conversion of the patient's remaining exercise tolerance into physical training potentials will be summarized below.

The Evaluation of Exercise Tolerance

When examining the necessary conditions for admission to a training program, the first things to be established are the minimum requirements. In view of the large number of patients who could be considered for such training groups, minimum requirements are needed for reasons of capacity alone. The cardiologic "maximum" requirements to evaluate the exercise tolerance of the patient that are sometimes suggested even include *coronary arteriography* to evaluate the exercise tolerance of the patient. In view of the large numbers involved, this requirement is clearly impossible. Information concerning the state of the vasculature is, of course, useful in determining the risks. In our group, where coronary arteriographic data were available, serious incidents within or without athletic activity occurred only in patients with three-vessel disease. This does still not justify coronary arteriography as an entrance requirement for athletic activity, since the increased risk exists outside athletic activity as well. The critical indication for arteriography is only to answer the question about the possibility or necessity of coronary bypass surgery.

The ability to withstand stress is the only true criterion for admission to a training program for any patient. For this reason the *stress test* assumes a central importance, besides the general physical examination. Additional cardiologic examinations, such as echocardiography, Holter monitoring, Swan-Ganz catheterization, etc., are generally not considered essential, and should be limited to the problem patient. This is particularly true for the *Swan-Ganz catheterization,* which is considered frequently as an essential component in the evaluation of the exercise tolerance of a patient. It is true that very high pulmonary artery pressure levels can be reached under exercise that cannot be detected by routine ergometric studies. On the other hand, this question must be asked: What is the significance of these high pressures? Frequently this rise in pressure is a manifestation of decreased myocardial compliance, as a consequence of scarring, and not a sign of myocardial failure. In this context, Roskamm (1978) suggests that for staging purposes, the behavior of the cardiac output must be considered, which is usually not done in practice. In our longitudinal studies, an increased high pulmonary artery pressure proved to be a very poor prognostic sign for complications both within and without athletic activity. Therefore, we consider this test indicated only when a specific question must be answered, e.g., can the patient be exposed to stress in the presence of a large post-infarct scar on the ECG, a large heart on x-ray, a suspicion of myocardial insufficiency under stress, questionable symptoms, etc.

The actual *performance of the stress test* presents a problem in cardiologic practice, since it is done quite differently by different investigators. Consequently the results are difficult to compare. The report that a patient has an exercise tolerance of 75 watts may mean very different things, depending on whether the test was performed in the sitting or standing position; if the starting load was 25 or 75 watts; or if the load levels had to be accomplished in 2, 4, or 6 minutes. In order to be able to achieve comparable techniques, the *German Association of Sportsphysicians* (Flöthner, 1981) and the *German Association for Cardiologic Prevention and Rehabilitation* recommended a protocol which starts with 25 watts and increases by the same amount every two minutes until one of the customary criteria for stopping is reached. The stress test should be performed in the sitting position.

A patient may be admitted to a *coronary artery activity club* when the following criteria are met: no evidence of cardiac insufficiency, no indication of a hemodynamically active aneurysm, and no additional valvular lesion, particularly no aortic valvular stenosis.

In the stress test a load of at least 1 watt/kg body weight, i.e., an average of 75 watts, should be tolerated without difficulty. At this level of load, there should be no evidence of any of the customary indications for stopping, e.g., subjective (angina) or objective (ST depression) indications of coronary insufficiency, dangerous rhythm disturbances, systolic blood pressure over 200 mm Hg, or evidence of myocardial failure under stress (onset of dyspnea).

The above contraindications, appearing under stress, can be disregarded if they can be eliminated by drug therapy. Great caution must be exercised if the radiogram reveals a significant *cardiac enlargement,* if determination of the cardiac volume gives a figure of more than 13 ml/ kg body weight, or if resting ECG reveals the presence of a particularly extensive infarct. In these cases at least a Swan-Ganz catheterization should be performed. According to the criteria of the "Hamburg Model," which we also follow in our practice, the consent of the patients personal physician is mandatory.

Patients who do not tolerate stress and who therefore do not meet the entrance criteria cannot have their cardiocirculatory system functionally improved by physical training. Nevertheless, even in these patients, improvements can be made in coordination and through the use of the beneficial psychologic effects that may be achieved by athletic activity. These patients are now admitted in increasing numbers into the low-performance groups. The numbers provided by the "Hamburg Model" indicate that about 40% of the surviving postinfarct patients are able to participate in a coronary training club. Of this group only about 40% can be motivated to participate. This means that 15% of the roughly 75,000 surviving postinfarct patients in the German Federal Republic (approximately 10,000 each year) could be admitted to the clubs. In view of the increasing importance of the coronary artery activity clubs, this number could increase significantly over the next few years.

This large number of patients who each year enter the ambulatory coronary activity clubs raises the question of the *affordable capacity.* In view of the number of patients who leave the clubs, there is a certain equilibrium. The "Hamburg Model," which had reached the saturation point, suggests that the appropriate ratio is one coronary artery activity club for every 50,000 persons. The number of patients in each club should not exceed 20, since a larger number would make adequate medical supervision impossible. The considerable organizational problems encountered in this area are well described in the summary review by Flöthner (1981).

The Implementation of Athletic Activity With Coronary Patients

Appropriate implementation of athletic activity requires that the trainer and *physical education teacher* be properly qualified. Lack of understanding that exercise therapy can be adapted to individual needs is one of the things that gives this idea a bad name. Pictures of high-performance athletic groups flutter in front of the eyes of many of those who deny the benefits of athletics for the cardiac patient. The *prescription of athletics* by a physician should be done in the same way as the prescription of drugs, namely on an individually graded basis. The dose is determined by the stress test. The table designed by Lagerstrøm (1975) (see Fig 5–1) indicates how each wattload on the bicycle ergometer can be converted into running speeds. If a patient develops repolarization disturbances at a 125-watt load, he can be exposed to only 100-watt loads. If this patient weighs 70 kg, he should be able to achieve a running speed of 110 m/minute. The maintenance of individual speeds, in spite of running with a group, can be taught through some educational device, such as the *"triangular run,"* introduced by Lagerstrøm. In this scheme the patients follow a triangular course of identical base but longer sides, so that the more highly able patient runs a longer distance in 1 minute than the less able, while both return to the starting point at the same time (Fig 5–5).

In this way every patient learns to keep his own speed, even though he is running in a group. Once the patient develops a feel for his speed, the triangle can be dispensed with, and the heart rate becomes the controlling factor.

This model represents only one example that shows how medical data concerning the exercise tolerance of the cardiac patient can be used in the practice of athletic therapy. The close cooperation between the physician and the physical educator in the care of the postinfarction patient is well demonstrated in this example. The physician sets the parameters that are then filled in by the physical educator. In this connection we must, once again, emphasize the importance of *controlled and measured physical exercise.* Using the patient to *count his own pulse* is frequently objected to for the following reasons: The pulse rate is a poor indicator for the assessment of the intensity of the load, because the patient frequently counts incorrectly, or because the pulse rate was influenced by drugs or the disease itself. Furthermore, the patient can be made into a neurotic by making him count his pulse all the time, and constantly reminding him of his underlying illness.

Practical experience leads us to a different conclusion. The regular "ritual" of counting the pulse reminds the patient, the athletic trainer, and the physician that this is not a general physical activity group, but a group of patients with serious cardiac problems. In spite of all neg-

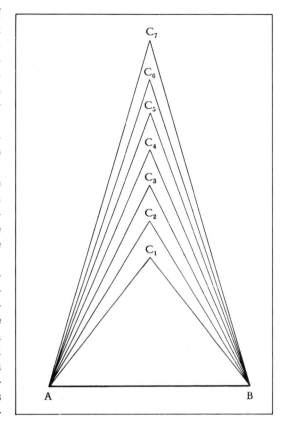

FIG 5–5.
Triangular run according to Lagerstrøm. This running method provides an educational technique that helps to overcome one of the fundamental problems of training in the framework of the coronary artery activity clubs. The individual patients should be given specific, individually tailored exercise and should not be forced to adapt to a group mean. The individual running speed can be taught on the basis of this triangular method. Each patient's exercise tolerance is determined by ergometric testing at approximately 100-watt load. This will be converted into running speed with the conversion table presented in Figure 5–1. The above indicated triangular running paths are marked with flags. All triangular runs should be completed in one minute and the individual runners are assigned to the different tracks according to their exercise tolerance. In this way each patient runs according to their individual speed, but still keeps up with the group. Once the patient has learned to stick to his/her individual speed, the triangular track can be dispensed with. The further control of maintaining the appropriate load intensity can be determined by pulse rate measurements.

ative value judgments, the pulse rate is the only practical measure for the intensity of load. The general, subjective impression that excessive stress may or may not be present would require a continuous medical supervision, which is impossible in practice. It has been our experience that in the groups in which the counting of the pulse was discouraged, random sampling of the patients revealed occasional severe overloading. As far as the limitations imposed on using the pulse rate by drugs and other causes are concerned, it is obvious that these must be taken into account when the patient's normal pulse frequency is established. In this context, reference must be made to the section on "Cardiac Drugs and Physical Exercise." In summary, we can conclude the discussion of the pulse rate as a control measure by paraphrasing Churchill's comment on democracy: "Pulse rate is certainly the worst measure of load intensity, but unfortunately there is no better one."

Evaluation of the Various Athletic Activities From the Point of View of the Coronary Patient

Running is certainly not the only form of exercise that can be recommended to patients. If one reviews the current literature to determine the forms of activity that are recommended for the coronary patient, one may come to the conclusion that only endurance exercises, such as running and ergometer-riding, are suitable. These recommendations are usually based on circulatory and metabolic studies, which suggest that only endurance loading will affect the circulation and the metabolism. On the other hand, the coronary patient should never be considered a simple heart-circulation-metabolism creature. The goals stated for athletic activity must be viewed from a holistic patient point of view. Athletic activity should never be directed only toward the cardiocirculatory system, but always toward the entire patient, both body and psyche. There are thus, on the other side of the ledger, programs for coronary artery patients that have an educational and psychologic orientation and in which there is practically no place for endurance exercises (see Hopf and Kaltenbach, 1977).

Between these extremes a reasonable middle road should be found. For this reason, in the athletic groups cared for by us, we offer a universal athletic program, which attempts, as much as possible, to affect the entire body and psyche of the patients. The center of this program is still, however, endurance training, since this is the only way in which significant therapeutic effects can be achieved on the cardiocirculatory function and on metabolic adaptation from the point of view of functional economy. This endurance training is supplemented with a gymnastics program that teaches coordination, mobility, and better muscular utilization, and with a play program that serves to abreact the stress factors in a psychic fashion, and that also serves to motivate toward participation in endurance activities.

Among the endurance activities, *running* was particularly emphasized initially since it has numerous advantages over similar forms of physical activity. Running requires minimal equipment in comparison to swimming, rowing, bicycle riding, or cross-country skiing. Running is particularly beneficial from a hemodynamic point of view, since it requires practically no forceful effort and yet utilizes almost all the muscle mass (see section on "Cardiac Work Under a Dynamic Load"). *Running* furthermore does not require extensive coordination. The ability to transform the watt-output, measured on the bicycle ergometer, into the speed of running, could not be done with swimming, since differences in technique of swimming would lead to significant differences in individual cardiocirculatory loads, even if the speed of swimming remains the same. Running fulfills the requirements best for a form of athletic activity that can be graded and controlled on an individual basis for all members of a group.

As an alternative to running, the other endurance activities can be used to a greater or lesser degree. Concerning the differences, particularly concerning the different effects on circulation, reference must be made to the section on "Heart Action Under Physical Exercise." The most important sports-medical considerations of the alternative endurance activity forms are summarized as follows: compared to running, *bicycle riding* has the disadvantage that it uses less of the total musculature, yet requires greater force. This, however, leads only to a slight increase in blood pressure. One of the advantages of bicycle riding is the fact that in this exercise the weight of the body is supported by the equipment. This is particularly helpful in the overweight person or in those who cannot run because of a skeletal disability such as arthritis.

Bicycle riding has a most important role in early cardiac rehabilitation in the form of *ergometer training.* On this equipment, it is possible to measure the amount of load exactly. In the later stages of rehabilitation, when the loss of performance, due to disease-induced lack of activity, has been corrected, such precise quantification of effort is no longer necessary. Riding an ergometer also becomes very boring after a while. The many questions from coronary patients and also from healthy persons as to what kind of ergometer to use can be answered by the statement that a sweat suit and running shoes make all such equipment unnecessary. Most of the ergometers purchased for exercise end their days in the basement, once their novelty has worn off. In addition, most of the inexpensive, *home exercisers* cannot be adjusted precisely and have an insufficient mass to make riding on them an enjoyable experience.

With very few exceptions, namely those for whom because of their severe load limitations, a very accurately determined training program is required, prescription of such equipment cannot be justified to the Public Health Insurance Fund even though many patients ask for them. There are very few patients who can organize their life with sufficient discipline, and who can maintain an ergometric training program regularly, over a longer period of time.

The following points must be emphasized for *swimming:* swimming, particularly in the context of rehabilitation for the postinfarction patient, is a subject of lively controversy. On the one hand, swimming is an ideal form of exercise from the point of view of sports medicine. It is one of the endurance sports and it can be performed, contrary to running, by overweight patients and those who have serious limitations in walking because of advanced arthritis. The weight of the body is supported, just as in bicycle riding, by the equipment, in this instance by the water. Against this positive value of swimming is the fact that there are a number of reports about serious incidents that occurred during swimming. Of 13 deaths during physical activity that occurred at the Hohenried Rehabilitation Clinic over a period of 10 years, 10 occurred during swimming (Halhuber, 1972). The cause is given as a vagal reflex, causing the so-called *diver bradycardia.* Samek (1978) observed surprising and serious arrhythmias by telemetry during swimming that could be attributed to this mechanism. Besides this mechanism, these deaths may well have had additional etiologic factors, such as increased venous return due to the hydrostatic pressure on the vessels in the skin, the occasional breath-holding, panic reactions, and overexertion due to uncontrolled stress.

These conditions should not lead to the conclusion, however, that swimming should be forbidden to all coronary patients. Patients with adequate myocardial reserves can be permitted to swim, although those with a known tendency for dangerous arrhythmias must be excluded. The diver bradycardia must always be considered when the load-intensity is being determined. The same pulse rate in swimming denotes a much higher load than in running. We advise our patients not to swim for at least 6 months after the infarct. There are, however, a number of rehabilitation centers where water exercises are used successfully in the framework of a broad rehabilitation program. This requires a very careful selection and supervision of the patients. In the later stages of rehabilitation, swimming can be recommended, provided that there is a sufficient cardiac reserve, without any sign of insufficiency (minimum 1 watt/kg body weight), and that there is no evidence of any significant rhythm disturbance. If swimming is performed in the framework of a supervised coronary artery activity club, it is mandatory that these patients be very carefully monitored by the instructors.

The *optimal water temperature* is given as 27° C. Colder water is undesirable, since in view of the relatively limited motion capability of the coronary artery patient, hypothermia is a very real danger. Swimming in very warm water, found in some spas, places a twofold circulatory demand on the patient by virtue of the need for thermoregulation, and is hence very undesirable. In connection with any discussion about the effects of water and temperature on the circulation of coronary patients, it behooves us to mention the catchword *sauna* since much information is needed on this subject. The rise in pressure after diving into water is particularly noticeable when the water is cold. Bachmann (1970) found increases in systolic pressure to 300 mm Hg. As discussed in detail in the section on "Arterial Pressure," this is largely the consequence of the superimposed water

pressure. The danger of sudden cooling is therefore not due to the hypertensive circulatory state, since this hypertensive state is largely due to the superimposed hydrostatic water pressure. The important and dangerous event for the cardiac patient is the *sudden autonomic stimulus.* It is a simultaneous, severe vagal and sympathetic stimulus. While the vagus primarily affects and slows the atria, the sympathetics activate the ventricular excitatory foci. This is the "ideal" situation to trigger ventricular fibrillation. For this reason the postinfarct patient should avoid jumping into cold water. The stimulus of cold water in the shower can be dangerous in the same way.

Both the *usefulness* and the dangers of the sauna in training are generally overestimated. The circulatory stress in the sauna is relatively small. The studies of Eisalo (1975) performed with dye-dilution techniques, showed an increase in cardiac output to 10 L/min and a simultaneous drop in peripheral resistance of 40%. This corresponds to a circulatory load of 75 watts, which is similar to the load of light jogging. This light load will not provide a training stimulus to the circulation. On the other hand, there is no reason why a postinfarct patient, who regularly participates in an athletic program, should not be allowed to use the sauna. A *condition* of this permission is, of course, that the patient will not jump into cold water from the sauna. Furthermore the patient should become used to the sauna slowly. He should not stay in the sauna room for more than 10 minutes and at a temperature of not more than 80–90° C. After the sauna a tepid shower or a slow swim in 24° to 27° C water is recommended. Since thermoregulation usually leads to hypotension after the sauna, a sufficient period of rest in the supine position must be included.

Following these precautions, we have encountered no problems with the sauna in patients after a myocardial infarct. As a cautionary measure, these patients should be advised not to use the sauna for about 6 months after their infarct. While the sauna has no direct effects on the training of the cardiocirculatory system, it is an excellent method to foster the ability of the patient to adapt to varying conditions. The rise in blood pressure due to the stimulation of cold water after the sauna is particularly useful in improving the regulatory mechanics of circulation in the patients with functional circulatory problems, e.g., hypotension and the orthostatic syndrome.

Rowing is a form of stress that, at least in its athletic form, is undesirable for coronary artery patients for several reasons. The hemodynamic disadvantages of the rhythmic, high intensity effort and the accompanying steep rise in blood pressure was discussed in the section on "Cardiac Function Under Physical Exercise." Even though rowing is a typical endurance activity, it is usually performed as a team effort and thus does not lend itself to the fundamental requirement of having individually adjusted and supervised loads. The coronary artery patient who rows in a four-man boat must keep to the same rate and rhythm of rowing as the other, frequently more physically capable team mates. Even if the rowing coronary artery patient does not fall into the water and thus trigger a ventricular fibrillation (this happens occasionally), rowing still raises a number of other concerns.

According to the above remarks, running is good, but rowing is bad. On the other hand, however, these examples illustrate the important point that in evaluating athletic activity for the cardiac patient qualitative considerations are less important than the quantitative ones. The occasionally dogmatically debated question about which athletic activity is good and which is bad is much less important than the one that asks: "In what form and to what extent is that particular athletic activity performed?" Thus, running is a sensible physical activity, but when it is done under high-performance conditions and under the motto of "Run the marathon after your infarct," then running is much more dangerous than a physical activity like sensibly-implemented rowing. The above-listed concerns about rowing can be dismissed if the rowing takes place in a wide-beamed, safe, single rower boat, and if the coronary patient can be convinced to avoid a high-effort performance and to limit himself to excursion-style, sensible rowing.

The last two endurance activity forms that must be mentioned in connection with the coronary artery patient are performed at *higher altitude*. These are mountain climbing and alpine skiing. In this context, coronary artery patients frequently ask, at what altitude is it safe for them to remain and/or engage in physical activity? Theoretically, the reserves contained in the oxygen dissociation curve allow the blood to be fully saturated at altitudes up to 2,000 m. Experience has shown us, however, that the ability to respond to stress becomes limited at much lower altitudes. In comparative studies, we have seen that under identical ergometric loads, the average pulse was 10 beats per minute higher, and repolarization disturbances occurred more frequently in a group of coronary artery patients doing cross-country skiing in the Black Forest (elevation 1,300 m), than in Cologne (elevation 50 m) (Fig 5–6).

This observation can possibly be explained by the frequency of pulmonary diffusion disturbances, which are present because of the heavy smoking history of the coronary artery patients. For this reason coronary patients should be advised not to engage in stressful activities at elevations over 1,000 m during the first year. The patient with good reserves may be allowed, after this period of time, to engage in athletics even at an altitude of 2,000 m, particularly after he has learned

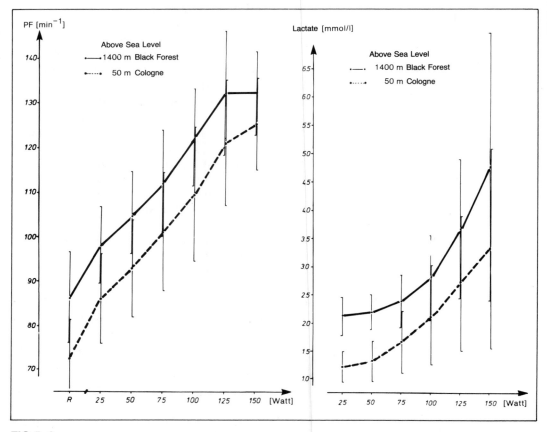

FIG 5–6.

Representation of the heart rate and serum lactate levels at equal loads determined in members of the Cologne coronary artery activity club, once in Cologne and once during a cross-country ski week on the Feldberg in the Black Forest (assembled by Jacob, in preparation). Even though the difference in altitude is not excessive, there is a distinct elevation in pulse rate and serum lactate at the higher altitude.

to monitor his own exercise activities. Halhuber (1981) formulated the very sound advice for these patients, namely, that they can remain at the so-called commercial altitudes, i.e., they can stay at any altitude at which there is a permanent commercial establishment. Activity at higher altitudes, e.g., mountain climbing, should not be recommended. While *hiking*, in general, has no training effect on the cardiocirculatory system, in view of its low load-intensity, *hiking in the mountains* may produce such an effect. In the healthy person, the criterion for effective load intensity is the achieve-

ment of a pulse rate of 180 minus the age in years. In the coronary artery patient this may have to be modified if drugs such as β-blockers have been prescribed.

Cross-country skiing has proven to be a highly effective form of exercise for the coronary patient. It is not, however, free of problems. This form of exercise can be considered to be ideal from a locomotion physiology point of view, since it requires very little muscular force, at least as long as it is performed on level ground. On the other hand, the muscle mass involved is very large. The use of the poles leads to the utilization of all four extremities that, in a way, simulates a walk on "all fours." The muscle mass used is even greater than in running. Technically, cross-country skiing can be learned easily by even those coronary patients who have never skied before, but who can learn quickly to move forward on skis. The danger of injury is very small, when compared to downhill skiing, since the rate of motion is slow and the bindings between the foot and the ski are loose. The high motivational effect of movement in a beautiful environment is very important.

It is precisely this point, however, that constitutes the first *disadvantage* of this athletic activity. The stimulation of moving in a beautiful environment tends to make people forget their personal limits. The temptation is great to fully immerse oneself into the skiing experience over a single weekend. The pressure to keep up with a group and to complete a cross-country course ignores the requirements for individually tailored exercise. There are also additional external factors such as change in climate, particularly cold weather, that may trigger "cold-angina." A factor that cannot be ignored is the friendly "après-ski" get-together, where the consumption of alcohol may assume dangerous proportions.

These disadvantages can explain why there are recurring reports concerning incidents during cross-country skiing. Even though our own experiences in the framework of the Cologne coronary artery activity club were positive, there were significantly more cardiac complications requiring intervention during cross-country skiing in comparison with other exercises. The two most important ones were one case of ventricular fibrillation and one case of reinfarction that occurred in a patient without appreciable physical activity. Cross-country skiing can be recommended to the coronary artery patients, but only after very careful preparation, limitation of the distances

covered, and monitoring the intensity of load by measuring the pulse rate.

In this connection, it seems logical to comment on the possibility of recommending *downhill skiing* to the coronary patient. This is an activity about which many questions are asked by patients. Basically, downhill skiing requires strength, mobility, and coordination. Arterial pressure measurements by Bachmann (1970) revealed significant increases in pressure. A training effect on the cardiocirculatory system cannot be expected. If one adds the high risk of injury, downhill skiing cannot be recommended for the coronary patient. A postinfarct patient should not try to learn this sport.

The situation is quite different in an experienced downhill skier who suffers a myocardial infarct. Here resumption of skiing may be permitted in the individual case. A precondition must be that the patient have sufficient cardiac reserves and a psychologic make-up that gives him sufficient self discipline to avoid overexertion. The possibility of injury in the enthusiastic downhill skier may affect the decision concerning *anticoagulant therapy*. Since the value of long-range anticoagulation is still debated, this may be a situation in which not to continue anticoagulant therapy. Practically the same considerations concerning circulatory load, training effects, and injury risks must be kept in mind as far as *horseback riding* and the coronary patient are concerned.

In view of the above discussion about the goals of treating coronary patients with athletic activities, serious consideration must also be given to calisthenics. Calisthenics affect primarily the motor functions, such as coordination, mobility, and muscular strength. Calisthenics can also be used in such a fashion to provide endurance training. *Improving coordination* is important for the coronary patient as well. It brings with it a greater economy in motion, which leads to better performance through greater efficiency, even in the patient with limited exercise tolerance. This is particularly meaningful in the context of the low-performance groups. The *improvement of mobility* has no direct effect on the cardiocirculatory system, but is still important for the coronary patient for general motor function. For the importance of calisthenics *developing strength,* the reader is referred to the section on "Work of the Heart Under Static Load."

Power-loading is fundamentally undesirable because of the resulting hypertension, and yet effective muscles are needed for all forms of motion. The smaller the muscle mass in the coronary patient, the greater the sympathetic drive that originates in the relatively overloaded muscles, even after a moderate load. Muscles are necessary for all forms of exercise, including endurance exercise and play exercises. For this reason all major muscle groups must be addressed in the framework of any calisthenic program. Naturally all such programs of strength development must remain at the lower end of the individual capacities, in order to avoid excessive hypertension. 50% of the maximal voluntary force is a reasonable goal to be achieved. Maximal powerloads—with their accompanying pressure response—must be strictly forbidden for reasons described in the section on "The Valsalva Mechanism."

In view of the greater rise in pressure under static loads, frequently all forms of submaximal power-loading are decried, often with very dogmatic statements. Such fears can be dismissed on the basis of the findings of Ferguson (1981), who reported a lower coronary artery perfusion at a 70% of maximal effort in manual grip-squeeze exercises than by bicycle ergometric work, which caused anginal pain in the same group of patients. In low-level static exercise the increase in oxygen requirement caused by the increase in blood pressure is bal-anced by a lesser increase in heart rate, when compared to the effects of dynamic exercise.

The only motor exercise form that should never be used in the coronary artery patient is *speed.* Speed exercises have no training effect on the cardiocirculatory system, are always associated with overloading it and, over time, with acidosis. In addition there is the danger of orthopedic injury through excessive stretching of the muscles and through tears of the muscle fibers, particularly in the older patients.

A separate discussion is required for the subject of *competitive games* and the coronary patient. On physiologic and pathophysiologic grounds competition should be forbidden, since it can lead to overexertion and to injury. This was expressed by Jahnecke (1974) for the hypertensive patient, although it applies even more to the postinfarct patient: "We forbid, as a matter of principle, all forms of athletics for our hypertensive patients, where, at the end there is a "winner" and a "loser" since only very rarely is pride a friend of common sense."

This point of view seems reasonable, when one considers the potentially harmful reactions for the cardiac patient that may be triggered by psychic stimulation. These are detailed in Figure 2–10. The possibility of producing dangerous rhythm disturbances must be emphasized. Stein (1976) had pointed out that psychic stimulation produced arrhythmias twice as frequently as physical exercise.

The same idea can also be supported with purely psychologic arguments. It can be argued that competition gives the postinfarct patient an opportunity to act out his A-type personality to the fullest, and in this he may even be further encouraged by an A-type sports physician. On the other hand, one should remember that man is not a "running animal," as is so dogmatically stated in the long-distance-running literature. The large majority of persons who come to a sports arena are turned on by competition. Man can be described therefore as *"Homo ludens,"* the playing (competing) man. Hüllemann (1974) called the "Heidelberg Model," that was the first one to be engaged scientifically with the coronary patient, the "ludens club."

The patient must be given an opportunity to get rid of the daily accumulation of psychologic stress factors during competition. Competitive games are also a good motivator to return and to continue to participate in physical activity. They provide the stimulus for the patient to accept the "medical necessity" of endurance exercises. Games can and should be made a part of all exercise programs for the postinfarct patient. It is an athletic-educational responsibility to make sure that the potentially harmful aspects and the overly prideful competing spirit be properly controlled.

This responsibility begins with the selection of competition play. It is consistent with the general principle governing coronary artery activity clubs to select team sports, rather than solo sports, since theoretically, the problems of the club can be better resolved in a group activity. Beyond this, single competitions like tennis are more likely to lead to overexertion, because there are fewer opportunities for rest. Unfortunately, the "game of games" in Germany is *soccer,* and therefore, this type of sport is sometimes chosen in the coronary artery activity clubs. Soccer is an excellent example of the team sport that should not be chosen for this purpose. The run after the ball can easily lead to overexertion, and collisions with opponents can lead to injury. It is well to remember that many coronary patients are on maintenance anticoagulant therapy. Similarly undesirable are team *handball* and *basketball.*

In contrast, the so-called "team-rebound games" in which the teams are separated by a barrier have proven very satisfactory. These games include: *volleyball, rush ball, prell ball* and *soccer-tennis* (a game similar to volleyball, in which the ball is kicked over the net), and, in a more limited way, *indiaka* and *fistball.* In these games the opposing teams are separated at all times by a net or barrier. The player next to each player is a team mate who must be protected and not an opponent who must be attacked. The ball-chasing distances are relatively short.

In addition, it is the responsibility of the athletic instructor to modify some of the rules and to adapt them to the needs of the postinfarct patient. In the clubs in Cologne, *volleyball* is the favorite form of activity. As is well known, in this sport the danger of injury at the net is considerable. For this reason, "smashes" and "body blocks" are forbidden, and so is running backward, since this frequently leads to injury. The requirement to handle the ball at least two or three times transforms the game from one of apartness to one of togetherness. It is particularly helpful, if there are more than the required six players, since this allows rotation and rest for each. This example also illustrates the very great responsibility that rests on the athletic instructor when physical training is being implemented in postinfarct patients. Using the modified rules described above, we have seen no serious circulatory complications and only relatively few injuries during the 10 years that we have used volleyball as a major activity in the coronary artery activity clubs in Cologne. Monitoring heart rates and lactate levels revealed that the circulatory and metabolic stresses in volleyball were consistently lower than those regularly seen in running.

A particularly frequently asked question by the athletically oriented coronary artery patients concerns their ability to play *tennis.* Tennis belongs to the so-called "*solo rebound*" games and must be considered together with the related athletic activities, such as table-tennis, badminton, and squash. Weber (1980), in our group, made a special study of this problem. His investigations showed, not unexpectedly, that the last two forms of athletic activity, *badminton* and *squash*, were generally undesirable for the postinfarct patient. Since the initial moves are learned relatively easily, it does not take long before the game is accelerated to the point where it leads to very high pulse rates and lactate levels.

Tennis and table tennis are different. Here, the beginner is unlikely to overexert himself for lack of technique. For *table tennis* our observations were that in this activity the older beginner rarely proceeds beyond the "ping-pong player" level. Table tennis can thus be considered a very suitable activity for the coronary artery activity clubs. This, of course, does not hold for the experienced table tennis player who has had an infarct. In the high-class, experienced table tennis player, this activity is associated with high cardiac and metabolic stress. For such patients the resumption of this activity cannot be permitted with a clear conscience.

Contrary to table tennis, *lawn tennis* is characterized by longer running distances. According to the above-mentioned studies by Weber, tennis leads to significant cardiac and metabolic stress rather rapidly, even in the beginner. For this reason this activity should not be recommended for the coronary patient. The problem is quite different in the enthusiastic, former tennis player who does not ask whether he can play tennis, but rather, whether he can resume his previous favorite activity. Permission to do so must depend on the evaluation of the individual case. If the infarct is old enough (on the average, 1 year) and if the individual can tolerate loads of 125 watts and more, permission may be granted. A further consideration must be the psychologic stability of the patient. A player who is known to get into a real dither over every lost point, and thus, practically invites the next infarct, clearly should not be permitted to set foot on the court. We advise patients who wish to take up tennis again after an infarct to stay away from competitions. We also believe that doubles are less stressful than singles particularly when played against weaker opponents. A very nice arrangement is to play in mixed doubles with one's spouse.

The Exercise Tolerance of the Coronary Patient After a Bypass Procedure or Aneurysmectomy

A question frequently encountered in practice concerns the ability of a patient to engage in physical conditioning after a *bypass operation*. This question will arise even more frequently in the future when this procedure becomes available to all coronary patients on an almost routine basis. It is obviously possible to assess the patient's ability to undergo physical stress on an individual basis, even after a bypass operation. The postbypass patients seem to constitute a group that is particularly well suited for training activities. The patients who have undergone a coronary bypass procedure are a select group of patients quite similar to those who participate in a coronary artery activity club. It is usually a group of younger patients. In the group reported by Walter (1982), 90% of the postbypass patients were under 60 years of age. One of the prerequisites for a successful cardiac revascularization is the presence of enough healthy functional myocardium. It can additionally be assumed that the patients who subject themselves to such an operation are ready to participate actively in the framework of an exercise group.

The coronary arteriography that precedes the operation and the intraoperative observations give optimal information concerning the cardiac status of the patient and concerning his exercise tolerance, which is usually improved as a result of the surgical procedure. As shown in the already quoted findings of Walter, the pulmonary wedge pressure becomes normal on a stress test in many patients. The total load that can be tolerated is frequently significantly improved postoperatively. These positive arguments can be substantiated by our own findings. Compared to the entire group of coronary heart disease patients monitored by us the postbypass group had a very low incidence of cardiac problems.

Another group of post cardiac surgery patients presents a much more difficult problem. These are the patients who have had an *aneurysmectomy*. According to the original guidelines used for admission to the coronary artery activity clubs in the "Hamburg Model," and that are still generally considered to be valid, the presence, or even the suspicion of the presence, of a hemodynamically active aneurysm was a definite contraindication for recommending physical activity for the postinfarct patient (Flöthner, 1981). The situation is quite different, however, if the cause of the contraindication, i.e., the aneurysm, had been surgically removed.

Nevertheless, it is important to caution against an oversimplified approach to this problem. Patients with an aneurysm are frequently more capable of withstanding stress than patients after an aneurysmectomy. This depends on the diagnostic criteria used for this operation. Patients after aneurysmectomy are a poor group to choose from. According to Blümchen (1980), most aneurysmectomies are performed because of serious, refractory arrhythmias or because of cardiac insufficiency at rest or under stress. Only rarely is this procedure performed purely on the basis that the aneurysm can be clearly circumscribed or that there is sufficient healthy, functional myocardium. Consequently, a comparison of a conservatively-treated group and a surgically-treated group showed a distinctly higher mortality in the latter group. Within an observation period of 42 months, only three of 27 conservatively-treated patients died, while during an observation period of only 11 months, there were four deaths in a group of 24 aneurysmectomized patients.

The presence of a relatively favorable prognosis in this apparently carefully selected and conservatively treated group of patients makes the arbitrary denial of admission of patients with an aneurysm into the coronary artery activity clubs a highly questionable process. Since 15% to 35% of all transmural myocardial infarcts lead to an aneurysm or myocardial dyskinesia (Carstens, 1982), it can be assumed that among the patients who were admitted to coronary artery activity clubs without invasive diagnostic studies, many have an unsuspected aneurysm. We have observed a number of cases in the group monitored by us where this diagnosis was made much later on the basis of a ventriculogram. The categorical denial of physical exercise for patients with an aneurysm was based on the belief that this could lead to an overload of the remaining myocardium by an increased volume which has to be pumped into the volume of the aneurysmal sack during exercise. On the other hand, such an occurrence was doubted on the basis of pathologic findings and in view of the decreased elasticity of the aneurysmal sack (Swan, 1976). It therefore seems justifiable to admit patients with aneurysms at least to the low performance group, provided they can tolerate increased stress.

The patient after an aneurysmectomy, in contrast to the nonoperated patient, must be considered to be a high-risk patient. Hemodynamic studies have shown that the operation does not necessarily result in a definite improvement in the hemodynamic behavior under stress. Even though certain authors report functional improvement in the left ventricle under stress, as measured by pulmonary artery pressure (Jehle, 1981), other authors assume that these are exceptional cases (Blümchen, 1981). In general the number of patients who are improved by the operation is about the same as the number who are made worse. Such variability in the surgical results can be attributed to the differences in surgical criteria (size of the aneurysm, one- or more vessel disease) and on the resectability of the aneurysm, as well as on the ability of the surgeon to revascularize the myocardium.

Although there are few objective indications that the aneurysm patient's performance levels are improved by the operation, most authors are in full agreement, that as a rule, and in spite of the absence of any objective evidence of greater exercise tolerance, the patient subjectively feels capable of better performance. Of 29 patients examined by Carstens after surgery, 10 claimed to be much better and 12, as better able to stand stress. This is a striking example of the difference between subjective feelings and objective findings.

Every patient must be evaluated individually and very carefully following an aneurysm resection, when considered for admission into a coronary artery activity club. Participation in a low performance group should be frequently possible. Participation in a general coronary artery activity club only rarely. Our own experience is limited to five cases, although two of these have been active in our athletic program for several years, and certainly seem to justify such a trial.

CARDIAC DEFECTS

The Exercise Tolerance in Patients With Cardiac Abnormalities

Exercise tolerance and the limits of permissible physical activity are quite different in patients with congenital and ac-

quired heart disease. The accidental discovery of a lesion is one of the most common events in sports medicine cardiology. It is astonishing how effective some athletes can be in spite of an existing lesion. The question about exercise tolerance must therefore always be answered after full consideration of the particular hemodynamic conditions. This is very significant in advising children with congenital defects concerning participation in school athletic activities. It is also becoming very important in the framework of cardiac rehabilitation after surgical correction of the lesion.

It is in connection with *school athletics* that the question of exercise tolerance is most frequently answered in the negative. The observation that children with congenital heart lesions are banned from all physical activity can unfortunately be made much too often. Yet, some smaller lesions, e.g., small ventricular septal defects, may leave the exercise tolerance virtually unimpaired. The hasty ban on all athletics is motivated either by thoughtlessness, or by over-protective parents, or by physicians and athletic instructors who are committed to think only in terms of safety. Even the observation that children are forbidden to engage in athletics because of a *functional heart murmur* is unfortunately not exceptional. One must remember that children can be damaged by this in several ways. It not only leads to a loss in overall fitness and joy of living, but it also deprives the child of social integration into a group.

An absolute ban on all physical activities can be justified only in very rare instances, and usually only on the basis of very severe multiple congenital defects. As rule, a *qualified ban on athletics* is sufficient, such as a ban on the most demanding forms of athletics, or a waiver from having to prove certain levels of achievement.

Even though such a classification can

be made only after the evaluation of the specific hemodynamic conditions on an individual basis, some general guidelines have been established by Jüngst (1977): In general, *pressure-related lesions*, e.g., valvular stenoses, are far more unfavorable for exercise tolerance than the *volume-related lesions*, e.g., shunts or valvular insufficiencies. This is due to the fact that volume-work demands considerably lower oxygen requirements than does pressure-work. Furthermore, pressure-related lesions are more likely to lead to massive cardiac hypertrophy, than do volume-related lesions. This in turn raises the danger of coronary insufficiency under exercise. Furthermore, the hemodynamic situation is likely to deteriorate in the pressure-related lesion, since the inevitable increase in cardiac output necessarily leads to an increase in the pressure gradient. The opposite is true in volume-related lesions, where a decrease in the peripheral resistance reduces the volume of the regurgitated blood, and thereby improves the hemodynamic situation.

Pulmonic stenosis must be mentioned prominently among the pressure-related lesions. If right ventricular pressure is less than 50 mm Hg, no significant reduction in exercise tolerance is to be expected. Nevertheless, and primarily on theoretical grounds, every child with this lesion should be forbidden to engage in any high performance athletic activity. Participation in other forms of school or association athletics may be permitted. If the pressure is between 50 and 100 mm Hg, some school athletic activity may be permitted, depending on the symptomatology of the child. The children should be excused from the more hemodynamically demanding forms of activity (endurance exercises, participation in peak achievement tests, etc.). In children with a right ventricular pressure above 100 mm Hg, any query concerning athletic activity would, naturally, receive a negative answer. In fact, these children are usually symptomatic at rest. Just as in all other cases, it would be very helpful in determining exercise tolerance if hemodynamic data from both rest and stress studies were available.

Aortic stenosis poses much more complex questions than pulmonary stenosis. For purposes of athletic evaluation it does not matter if the stenosis is valvular, supravalvular, or subvalvular. Recommendations concerning exercise tolerance must be made particularly carefully in this situation, since sudden death can occur not infrequently under physical exercise in this disease. For this reason, in some centers, all physical activity is forbidden for these patients as a matter of general philosophy.

We consider this approach questionable in asymptomatic children who appear to have no limitations in performance and in athletes who started their training prior to discovery of the lesion. Our feelings on this subject are based on the general considerations discussed in some detail earlier. In opposition to this feeling, it can be said that the mortality statistics, discussed above in the section on "Sport Related Risks for the Heart," show aortic stenosis rarely, except as a component of obstructive hypertrophic cardiomyopathy. In addition, there are a number of aortic stenosis patients who are capable of astonishing exertions. In patients with aortic stenosis, all forms of high-performance athletics should be forbidden. Participation in school athletics may be considered on the same terms as those discussed for pulmonary stenosis, provided that there is good exercise tolerance, an unremarkable stress ECG, and careful medical supervision.

In *coarctation of the aorta* surgical correction is usually possible, or there may well be sufficient collateral circulation. The determinant factor in children is the blood pressure, which can rise to alarming levels under physical exercise.

Such pressure overshoots can be seen in children with this lesion, even after surgical correction (Madu, 1982). For this reason, athletic activities that require great pressure loads should be forbidden (heavy athletics, wrestling).

The *ventricular septal defect* is the most frequently encountered volume-related lesion. In very small septal defects, such as the already mentioned *maladie de Roger* the intensity of the murmur is inversely proportional to the hemodynamic significance of the defect. According to Jüngst (1977), and assuming careful cardiologic evaluation, even performance athletics can be permitted for selected individuals with this condition. Nevertheless, these patients should be advised to abstain from those athletic activities that are most demanding on the circulation. They should also be advised that they are, at least theoretically, at an increased risk.

Even in the presence of larger ventricular and atrial shunts participation in school athletics may be permitted, provided that the shunt is a pure *left-to-right* one and that the above-mentioned restrictions are observed. Exercise tolerance will be markedly affected if there is an increase in pulmonary artery pressure leading to a *right-to-left shunt*. In this situation the exercise tolerance has to be determined on an individual basis. The same considerations apply to a patient with a *patent ductus arteriosus*. A *right-to-left* shunt is present, by definition, in a number of the complex congenital lesions. The most common of these is the *tetralogy of Fallot*. In the latter case, the shunt is explained by the combination of the septal defect and pulmonic stenosis. Physical exercise will result in an increase in the right-to-left shunt. If this condition has not been repaired surgically by the time the child reaches school age, the child will spontaneously avoid any physical stress. These children must, naturally, be excused from all school athletic activities.

Exercise Tolerance in the Patient With Cardiac Lesions After Surgical Correction of the Defect

In determining the exercise tolerance of a patient after surgical correction of the cardiac defect, the nature of the lesion, the duration of the lesion, and the degree of which normal hemodynamic conditions have been reestablished must all be considered. In the ideal case, e.g., after closure of a small septal defect, it can be assumed that normal circulatory dynamics have been established and that the patient has a normal exercise tolerance. The situation may be different and new questions may be asked in view of the increasing success of valvular surgery, particularly in the older individual. The question of to what extent these patients can be exposed to physical exercise in the framework of a rehabilitation program cannot be answered yet, since there are only insufficient data on which to base a response. A patient following *valvular surgery* cannot be considered to be cured and healthy, as this is frequently, though erroneously, assumed. In these patients the range of activity continues to be limited. The data in the literature concerning exercise tolerance after valvular surgery range over a wide area. The exercise tolerance is much better in patients after aortic valve replacement than after mitral valve replacement. Mattern (1979) found that 59% of the former had a normal exercise tolerance, while only 24% of the mitral valve replacement patients and 22% of the double valve replacement patients have such normal tolerance.

Carstens (1981) is critical of the fact that most of the statistics rely on the patients' subjective reports, most of whom were improved by one or two New York Heart Association classes. Just as in the aneurysmectomized patient, this group shows a marked discrepancy between their subjective improvement and the clinically-proved objective improvement. Seventeen of the 35 patients in the author's series reported good to very good exercise tolerance and a distinct improvement. Yet a 50% increase in performance could be observed in only nine patients. In this group the best improvement was also found after aortic valve replacement.

The reasons for the limited exercise tolerance in patients after valve replacement are manifold. Partly this is the consequence of long-standing disease that had led to irreversible myocardial damage and to rhythm disturbances through chronic pressure- and volume-overload and increased myocardial stress. Further complicating factors include: intraoperative and postoperative cardiac damage, such as atrioventricular (AV) blocks, myocardial infarcts, and valve failure. Even after valve replacement, many patients show atrial fibrillation. Other causes include the multisystem diseases of old age, including coronary artery disease, present in so many of the elderly.

Another definite cause for the limitation of performance is the fact that, to date, the valvular prostheses are not perfect and by no means replace the normal valve. After replacing the aortic valve with a disc prosthesis, Forman (1978) reported a resting gradient of 7–35 mm Hg, which rose to 10–43 mm Hg under stress and in an extreme case even as high as 75 mm Hg. After mitral valve replacement, the resting pressure gradient was 12 mm Hg, which rose to 18 mm Hg under stress. These values correspond to a moderately severe aortic or mitral stenosis.

Stress conditions will thus demonstrate the presence of a pathologic hemodynamic status in the patients after valve replacement. Hemodynamic studies show the same thing. And yet it can be assumed that the hemodynamic limitations are smaller if the replacement has taken place because of an aortic lesion or a valvular stenosis than if it has taken place because of a mitral lesion or a valvular regurgitation. This was demonstrated by

Kraus (1982) with hemodynamic studies at rest and under stress. In this study, 20% of the patients with previous aortic insufficiency, 50% with previous aortic stenosis, and practically all patients following a mitral valve replacement, showed evidence of hemodynamic pathology. In the patients with aortic valvular lesions, this meant a pathologic rise in pulmonary artery pressure under stress, and in half of the above-mentioned patients, an inadequate rise in cardiac output. In the patients with mitral valve insufficiency, the hemodynamic situation was somewhat better than in the former stenosis patients, since in the insufficiency patients the resting pulmonary artery pressure was usually normal while in the stenosis patients 50% showed an elevated pulmonary artery pressure at rest. An inadequate rise in cardiac output was noted in 70% of the former mitral insufficiency patients and in 90% of the former mitral stenosis patients.

That physical exercise affects the hemodynamic status of post-mitral valve replacement patients unfavorably, even during daily activities, was shown by Bachmann (1970). He found in patients with mitral valve lesions an increase in pulmonary artery pressure, up to 72/24 mm Hg, i.e., significant pulmonary hypertension, even after climbing only one flight of stairs. In patients with aortic valvular lesions, the pressure did not change.

These data raise a serious concern of whether or not patients after valve replacement should ever be exposed to physical activity. In spite of these data, from a cardiologic point of view it seems perfectly permissible to recommend a sensible physical exercise program to suitable patients (Carstens, 1981; Kraus, 1982; Rothlin, 1982). Carstens raises the question if the limitations in performance in patients after valve replacement may not be due to the preceding long-term inactivity. The institution of physical activity certainly requires careful cardiologic monitoring. Information concerning the hemodynamic status at rest and under stress obtained by Swan-Ganz catheterization is an absolute requirement. Another question that must be asked is whether a temporary pulmonary artery pressure increase under stress has any negative effect on longevity. In spite of the superior hemodynamic performance data after aortic valve replacement, the statistics of Blömer (1980) show no difference in the survival rates of these patients, when compared with patients who had a mitral valve replacement.

The question of whether physical training has a negative or positive effect on patients who had valvular replacement will be answered only after long-range studies. Basic theoretic principles suggest, however, that endurance training is not appropriate for these patients. Even in these patients, however, it is desirable to design a program that aims to improve the economy of the cardiocirculatory function. On the other hand, the existing pressure gradient must be considered. Endurance training could negate the efforts to achieve a desirable reduction of the preexisting cardiac hypertrophy.

For this reason we assign these patients, in the framework of the coronary artery clubs under our supervision, only to low performance groups that undergo no endurance training, and where physical activity is limited to calisthenics and games.

Another perspective from which the physical activity in these patients must be considered is *anticoagulation*. Except in patients who had a bioprostheses inserted, ongoing anticoagulant therapy is absolutely essential because of the serious danger of clot formation on the artificial leaflet valves. It is critical that the athletic instructor do everything in his power to protect these patients from physical injury, since trauma may force the discontinuation of anticoagulant ther-

apy, which in turn may have disastrous results. Our own experiences with about 20 patients of this type over a period of three years have been very positive. An initial review of these patients suggests that exercise tolerance in the valve patients is significantly less than in the postinfarct patient, and that their "dropout" rate is considerably higher. On the other hand, we have had no serious problems with these patients during athletic activities.

MYOCARDITIS, CARDIOMYOPATHIES

As described in the section on "Sport Related Risk for the Heart," myocarditis and cardiomyopathy, particularly of the hypertrophic kind, are among the most important causes of sudden death, even in young, apparently healthy athletes. Myocarditis may accompany seemingly minor infections and even localized sepsis. In *acute myocarditis*, all physical activity is contraindicated as a matter of course. In athletes, the appearance of previously unobserved arrhythmias should raise the suspicion of myocarditis. In this situation a thorough search for an infective focus is indicated (teeth, tonsils, sinuses). If acute myocarditis is a probable diagnosis, we will not allow any physical activity for at least 6 months, and even then only after a satisfactory stress ECG. A patient with old, chronic myocarditis should be evaluated in exactly the same way as a patient after a coronary infarction.

Reliable information concerning the exercise tolerance of patients with *cardiomyopathy* is lacking. The observation that patients with hypertrophic cardiomyopathy sometimes die under physical stress has led to the feeling that all physical activity should be forbidden for these patients. This certainly does not seem to be justified. In the individual case, such a decision should be made only on the basis of the type and extent of the disease. In significant *hypertrophic cardiomyopathy*, physical activity should be forbidden particularly if the myopathy has an obstructive component.

The same is true for the *dilational or congestive cardiomyopathy.* In the milder cases such an absolute ban is not desirable. Kuhn (1980) even recognizes a latent form of myopathy in which the ventricular volume and the thickness of the myocardium are normal. This type of a problem should be considered in an athlete who suddenly develops a repolarization disturbance on the resting or stress ECG in the absence of any previous coronary artery disease. Occasionally the diagnosis of cardiomyopathy can be made only by a myocardial biopsy.

In cases of a *latent cardiomyopathy,* or a mild, nonobstructive hypertrophic form of myopathy, physical exercises may be permitted, but only under careful cardiologic monitoring. Performance sports, or activity to the limits of endurance, should be discouraged in all cases. We also recommend that these patients abstain from all endurance activity since such activity could, at least in theory, increase hypertrophy, and in the congestive form of the disease, dilatation. This was discussed in the section on "Echocardiographic Findings." All pronounced-effort exercises should also be avoided, because of the negative effects of the Valsalva maneuver and the possibility of aggravating a concentric hypertrophy. This leaves only calisthenics and game sports for these patients, just as it does for the coronary patients.

ARRHYTHMIAS, HEART BLOCK, AND PACEMAKER PATIENTS

Disturbances in impulse generation and conduction are a part of most of the cardiac problems discussed above. They were also mentioned in connection with the findings in the athlete's heart ECG. Nevertheless, they will be briefly discussed again, since in practice they raise many questions that are independent of the underlying disease, and since arrhythmias can occur in the absence of any detectable organic lesions. Obviously, in all cases a serious attempt should be made to discover an underlying pathologic process, and if possible, provide appropriate clinical therapy. Unfortunately it is never possible to predict with any certainty whether any particular antiarrhythmic drug will produce the required antiarrhythmic effect in any given individual. If there are arrhythmias that occur during stress and that require therapy, then the effects of the therapy must be tested under stress conditions by ergometry or by Holter monitoring.

The most important *arrhythmias* occurring under stress are the *premature beats*. Single, unifocal atrial or ventricular premature beats require no treatment. When they are first observed in an otherwise healthy athlete, they should trigger a search for an inflammatory focus (see section on "Myocarditis, Cardiomyopathy"). In contrast, multifocal, coupled (bigemini), or runs of premature beats must be treated before physical exercise can be permitted. Arrhythmias that occur in sudden attacks, e.g., *paroxysmal tachycardia* or *atrial fibrillation*, are discussed in the section on "Electrocardiographic Findings."

Patients with persistent *atrial fibrillation* need not be excluded from all athletic activity as a matter of course. In patients after valvular surgery, persistent arrhythmias are common. In these cases exercise tolerance must be determined by exercise tests. Basically, this depends on the pulse rate increase under load conditions. We frequently find significant increases in heart rate that are not due to cardiac insufficiency but to rhythm disturbances. An attempt should be made to control this rate increase through appropriate antiarrhythmic management, particularly full digitalization. Digitoxin, more effective in controlling heart rate, is preferable over digoxin. If the rate is not too great, these patients will have a surprisingly good exercise tolerance in spite of the lack of coordination between the action of the atria and the ventricles.

By contrast, in *atrial flutter,* physical exercise must be avoided until this rhythm disturbance is corrected. It is interesting to note that in this condition the heart rate will increase under increasing load only to a certain level and then remain constant, in spite of the continued rise in load. This is due to the fact that while at rest flutter waves are transmitted in an irregular fashion; under load this transmission will occur on a fixed 3:1 or 4:1 ratio.

Disturbances in conduction must be discussed in the order of the propagation of the impulse. Concerning exercise tolerance in the *sick sinus syndrome* and the occurrence of athlete's heart bradycardia, the reader is referred to the section on "Function of the Athlete's Heart at Rest." In these patients exercise tolerance will depend on the extent to which the heart rate can increase further under load conditions. This must be determined by a stress test. These patients should be advised not to participate in endurance activities, since the increased vagal tone will be functionally superimposed on and aggravate the symptoms of the sick sinus syndrome.

In contrast, the patients in whom the ECG shows a *bundle-branch block* have good exercise tolerance if there is no underlying pathology. This finding is not uncommon on routine examination in mass sport participants. If a stress ECG shows no major problem, these patients can be allowed to continue their activities. Care must be taken that the repolarization disturbances seen on the stress ECG not be interpreted as an additional coronary artery insufficiency. Needless to say, a bundle-branch block always de-

notes a cardiac lesion and thus high performance athletics must always be discouraged in these patients.

The *bifascicular block,* which is usually a combination of a left anterior hemiblock and a right bundle-branch block, is not necessarily a contraindication to participation in physical activity. We have encountered this defect in mass sport participants, who with this finding on the ECG practiced athletics for years without any problems. The permission to allow continued participation in athletics depends on the stress ECG. If the conduction time is normal at rest, and if under load conditions it is not prolonged in the face of increased heart rate, participation in athletics may continue if good cardiologic monitoring is provided.

Concerning a *complete AV block,* the reader is referred to the section on "Electrocardiographic Findings." It can be said briefly that the exercise tolerance in a complete AV block has to be evaluated with a stress ECG. Even here, physical exercise is not necessarily excluded. In case of the heart blocks, which have their onset at a very early age, a usually supraventricular subsidiary center is in a position to produce fast cardiac rates. It happens though, usually in the older patient with an AV block, that an insufficient ability to increase the heart rate leads to the appearance of dangerous arrhythmias. At this point, physical activity can no longer be recommended. Because of the increased vagal tone in endurance athletics, this activity should be discouraged in the patient with a third degree heart block, just as much as in the patient with a sinoatrial (SA) block, even though exercise tolerance may be good. Naturally, patients in whom a Stokes-Adams attack is a possibility must be advised against participation in flying, mountain climbing, swimming, and all other activities in which such an attack could be disastrous.

Recently, Jüngst drew attention to a special form of conduction disturbance that is of great importance in physical activity, particularly in the child and adolescent. This is the prolonged QT interval, as part of the *Romano-Ward syndrome*. In this condition, physical exercise can lead to syncopal attacks. Apparently the prolongation of the conduction process facilitates the appearance of dangerous tachyarrhythmias. In this context, reference is made to the discussion concerning the potential dangers inherent in training-adaptation. Even in the trained person, a prolongation of the QT interval beyond the norm can be observed. The arrhythmias that could potentially result from this and that could endanger the athlete have not been demonstrated to date (see Keren, 1981, and the section on "Historical Overview and Evaluation"). When syncopal attacks are reported in relatively untrained children and adolescents with a definitely prolonged QT interval, the possibility of this syndrome must be considered. In these cases a stress ECG and Holter monitoring must be done in order to study the QT interval. According to Jüngst (1983) in the case of the QT syndrome, the QT interval corrected for rate (QTc) does not become shorter with increasing load (Fig 5–7).

Finally, we must look at a question that is frequently asked in practice, namely, the question of the potential exercise tolerance in patients with implanted *pacemakers*. In the context of athletic exercises, this question is relatively rarely asked, since most of these patients are elderly and because the interest in athletic activity is much less in this group than in the coronary artery group in which participation in physical training is taken for granted.

Exercise tolerance in the pacemaker patient depends less on the pacemaker used than on the underlying disease and on the reaction of the patient to stress. The exercise tolerance must be studied very carefully in each individual patient and must include a stress test. All the

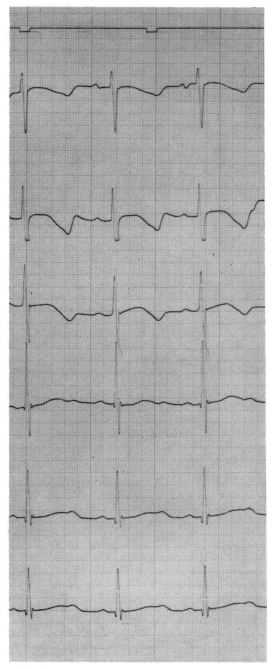

FIG 5–7.
Example of an electrocardiogram (ECG) showing the QT syndrome. The ECG was taken on a 7-year-old boy who had one episode of ventricular fibrillation and an episode of a questionable syncopal attack (chest leads are shown). The QT interval is clearly prolonged at 0.42 seconds.

factors listed above must be carefully considered.

When considering the underlying disease, one must realize that in some patients on pacemakers, an arrhythmia is dominant, while in others a myocardial component may be more significant. In those patients in whom the pacemaker was implanted primarily because of arrhythmias, the functional myocardial reserve may be subjected to considerably greater loads. The situation is quite different in patients in whom the pacemaker was implanted to improve myocardial function because of a bradycardic form of myocardial insufficiency. Arrhythmic and myocardial components can, of course, co-exist in the same patients.

A determinant factor may well be the ability to adapt the heart rate to changing load conditions. In many patients the pacemaker serves only as back-up insurance, and in these a sufficient increase in sinus rate is possible under varying load conditions. The exercise tolerance is far worse in patients who are limited even under exercise to a fixed pacemaker rate of 72 beats per minute. It is particularly unfavorable when in such patients the heart tries to compensate for inadequate rate increase by developing multifocal premature beats or runs of such beats. This would be similar to the situation described above in the patient with a complete AV block. Such response is seen with alarming frequency in pacemaker patients on a *stress ECG*. It is therefore surprising how rarely such tests are performed on pacemaker patients. The investigator frequently limits his studies to a "cosmetically satisfactory" resting ECG while ignoring the fact that in the pacemaker patient even the minor stresses of daily living, e.g., climbing one flight of stairs, may lead to dangerous arrhythmias.

In patients whose own rate cannot override the pacemaker under load conditions, athletic activity must be discouraged, since in these patients persistant overload of the stroke volume may lead to a highly undesirable dilatation of the heart. The arrhythmias that occur in these patients under load-conditions must be treated with antiarrhythmic drugs, if these arrhythmias appear to be life-threatening. If the arrhythmias occur only under severe load conditions, a stress test will determine the pulse frequency below which the patient can safely engage in physical activity.

As far as the type of pacemaker is concerned, selection falls in a very large percentage of all cases on the so-called "demand" pacemaker, which is triggered on demand by a probe located in the right ventricle (a more recent nomenclature defines these as type VVI). This type of stimulation is hemodynamically undesirable, since it does not provide for any cooperation between the atrium and ventricle. In this situation it also happens frequently that through retrograde stimulation the atrium contracts against the closed valves. For this reason, and particularly from the perspective of physical exercise, the so-called "sequential" pacemaker is hemodynamically much more satisfactory (type DDD). This pacemaker has an additional atrial probe so that each ventricular contraction is preceded by an atrial contraction.

On the other hand, it would be a euphemism, from the perspective of physical exercise, to speak about a physiologic type of impulse generation. The adaptation of cardiac action to physical load presumes appropriate sinus nodal function that is not present in many pacemaker patients, particularly in patients with the sick sinus syndrome. A patient with a ventricle-driven pacemaker in whom the sinus rate and the AV conduction increase appropriately under physical load is generally a much better candidate for physical exercise than the patient with so-called *physiologic stimulation* in whom exercise does not result in an appropriate rise in frequency.

Before recommending physical activity, it is essential to learn how the probes are anchored in the heart and what the consequences may be in case of a sudden pacemaker failure. In patients in whom the pacemaker was implanted recently, it can be assumed that a dislocation of the probe by myocardial twisting is not going to occur. Even in those patients, however, whose tolerance would ordinarily permit physical activity, those forms of athletics that involve violent arm motions must be discouraged. If the pacemaker has been implanted on the right side, a right-handed person should not play tennis, since this could lead to a dislocation of the pacemaker leads or cause some damage to them. Far more desirable for the pacemaker patient are those forms of activity that use mostly the legs. These include such activities as running and bicycle riding. It is obvious that all activities that may damage the pacemaker must be strongly discouraged. We know of one case where a blow during a boxing bout instantaneously disconnected the pacemaker. We advise all pacemaker patients to abstain from all those activities where, as in case of major arrhythmias, immediate professional assistance is not available. These include such activities as flying, mountain climbing, and diving.

6

Physical Stress and Cardiac Medications

The sparing effects of physical training on cardiac work compare favorably with the proven effects of beta blockers, and can thus no longer be doubted. This begs the question: why not use beta blockers in the first place? They are cheaper than gyms and safer than athletic activities.

Comments made in a discussion at the First International Congress on Cardiac Rehabilitation, Hamburg, 1977.

In the previous section we have tried to emphasize the great importance that today is assigned to physical exercise in cardiac patients. This importance makes it mandatory that the value of training be compared with other treatment modalities such as pharmacologic therapy and surgical measures.

It must be emphasized as vigorously as possible that exercise therapy and pharmacologic treatment should not be viewed as alternative measures. Athletics cannot replace drug therapy and neither can drugs achieve the kind of goals that can be reached with physical activity. This misconception is common among patients, who believe that physical exercise will eliminate the need for pills. On the other hand there are dyed-in-the-wool antisports physicians who represent the view that drugs can better and cheaper achieve the same goals as athletics. This view is illustrated at the beginning of this chapter in the quote, "Beta blockers are cheaper than gyms."

The improvement in physical fitness and psychologic well-being that results from athletics cannot be achieved with drugs and neither can the results of drug therapy be duplicated with physical activity. Physical activity and drugs should be viewed as separate processes that in the hands of an experienced and knowledgeable physician complement each other perfectly.

On the other hand, the relationships between drugs and athletics raise a number of interesting questions, in view of the manifold interactions between the effects of pharmacologic and exercise therapy. In the final analysis, the effects of physical training can be viewed as though they were drug effects. Knipping (1961) was the first to suggest that as a therapeutic measure, conditioning should be handled the same way as pharmacotherapy. Administered in the proper dose, it can be very helpful. In overdoses it can be harmful. "Underdosing" with physical training is just as useless as underdosing with drugs. Just as there are interactions between drugs, there are interactions between physical activity and drugs.

To give an idea about the variety of drugs taken regularly, even by the patient with good exercise tolerance, we list in Figure 6–1 the drugs taken by 166 postinfarct patients who were regular participants in athletic activities in our coronary artery activity club in Cologne in 1979. Indicating the year of this finding is important, since the spectrum of drug therapy is constantly in flux. On the average, each of the above patients who had relatively good exercise tolerance took three to four different medicaments. This question must be asked: "To what degree do these drugs modify the exercise tolerance of the patient?" In principle, the possible interaction between drugs and athletics can be classified as follows.

1. *Alterations in exercise tolerance.* This alteration in exercise tolerance can be either negative or positive.

2. *Alterations in the load-dependent reactions.* The advice of Knipping (1961) concerning the precise "dosing" of physical exercise in the cardiac patient makes it necessary to monitor the "dose" of exercise accordingly. In a sports-medical practice, the heart rate is the most important monitoring tool available. Heart rate is affected by a number of drugs, particularly by the beta-blockers. Beside the heart rate, drugs also modify other autonomic reactions, such as sweating, respiratory rate, skin perfusion, and the subjective feeling of exercise capacity. Even objective findings are modified by drugs, e.g., the stress ECG under the influence of digitalis.

3. *The reciprocal effects of drugs and physical activity.* Drugs and athletics can act synergistically or antagonistically. The β-blockers can again serve as examples. *The synergistic effects* are already evident from the indications for their use. Both are recommended for patients with coronary artery disease, the hyperkinetic heart syndrome, and hypertension. Strengthening the vagal effects on the heart is considererd to be the mechanism of action in both. *The antagonistic effects* are manifested by a limitation in exercise tolerance produced by β-blockers, at least in the healthy person, while exercise improves such performance. Antagonistic effects can also be seen in such areas as

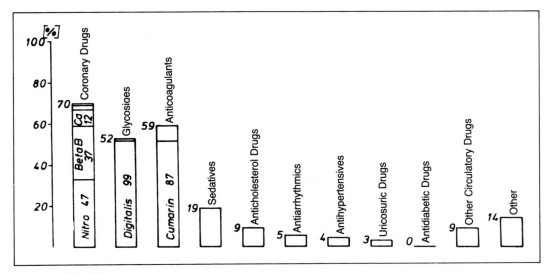

FIG 6–1.
Summary of the medications taken in 1979 by 166 patients in the Cologne coronary artery activity club (after Matschuk, 1982).

fat metabolism. In maintenance therapy the β-blockers raise the level of triglycerides and lower the level of the HDL-cholesterol, while exercise has the opposite effect.

THE BETA ADRENERGIC BLOCKING DRUGS

As already indicated in the general introduction to this section, the β-blockers have a particularly important place in a study of the relationships between drugs and athletics. Since physical activity accomplishes its effects on increased energy production and improved cardiocirculatory function by increasing the sympathetic stimulation, any substance that blocks sympathetic activity will have particularly drastic effects during physical load conditions. Some special aspects of the spectrum of the β-blockers activity can be particularly well demonstrated under load conditions. For this reason there are a large number of studies dealing with the problem of exercise tolerance under β-blockade. It seems justifiable, therefore, to devote a separate section to these drugs. In this section particular attention will be paid to the relationships between the drugs and athletics.

The great importance of the reciprocity between the effects of the β-blockers and of physical activity evolves in practice from the already-mentioned fact that there is a wide-ranging *analogy of effect* between the two. Both agents, β-blockers and athletics, produce a sparing of cardiocirculatory function that is manifested as a decrease in heart rate and contractility, and therefore a decrease in myocardial oxygen requirements, under identical load conditions. Beta-blockers and physical training are thus both used in organic cardiocirculatory diseases, i.e., coronary artery disease, hypertension, and arrhythmias, as well as in purely functional cardiac problems such as the hyperkinetic heart syndrome. It is therefore to be expected that β-blockers and physical training will be instituted simultaneously in the same patient. The question to be raised is, "To what extent is it indicated or contraindicated to recommend athletics to the β-blocked patient or to prescribe β-blockers to the patient who regularly engages in athletics?"

The analogy of effect between β-blockers and athletics can be seen particularly well when comparing the efficiency of the athlete's heart with the heart under β-blockade. This was discussed in detail in the section on "Function of the Athlete's Heart Under Physical Exercise." On the other hand, it must again be pointed out that in contrast to physical training, which raises the range of performance of the heart, β-blockers decrease this range of performance.

In any discussion concerning the effects of β-blockers on performance, a distinction must be made between the fields of *high performance athletics,* mass athletics, and cardiac rehabilitation. For the high performance athlete the potential negative or positive aspects of β-blockers depend on the particular form of athletic activity engaged in. It is well known that in athletic activities where performance depends primarily on psychologic factors, β-blockers are taken to improve performance. In athletic endeavours such as shooting, ski jumping, auto racing, flying, parachute jumping, and golf, β-blockers are taken allegedly, or really, to suppress the bothersome tachycardia and the occasional tremors. As is also well known, the consumption of pharmaceutic substances in order to improve performance is considered illegal *doping.*

Yet, at the time of preparing the translation of the manuscript for this monograph, the β-blockers have already been added to the list of the forbidden, *doping* drugs. This presents a problem for several reasons, including the fact that to date there is no evidence that β-blockers increase performance. To really prove this point it would be necessary to perform a controlled trial under the stress of world competition, e.g., national and international tournaments should be performed under double-blind, placebo-controlled test conditions. It is possible that in this area there are also great individual variations. It can be expected that some athletes are totally dependent on maximal psychologic stimulation for optimal results, while in others such a stressful situation will have negative effects. It is only this latter group in whom β-blockers may be helpful at least in theory.

The use of β-blockers in raising performance creates another area of controversy, since contrary to almost all other doping drugs, the β-blockers may have legitimate *indications* in the young athlete. These conditions would include hypertension or potentially threatening arrhythmias. It is particularly in the young hypertensive patient that β-blockers are the drugs of choice. It would be ethically indefensible to deny the use of β-blockers to a hypertensive rifle competitor purely on the basis of his athletic activities.

The situation is quite different in those forms of athletics where high energy outputs are required. It must be also said, however, that the data are presently insufficient to evaluate all forms of athletics. This is particularly true for those athletic activities in which only short bursts of energy are required and in which the energy supply contained in the high energy phosphates is sufficient (anaerobic energy metabolism). There is no evidence to date that would suggest a negative effect on this form of energy metabolism. Leaving the ethical considerations aside, there is at least theoretically no medical contraindication to the use of β-blockers under the competitive stress of *high jump, long jump, shot put,* and *weight lifting.* In view of the enormous increase in blood pressure under

strength-exercises, as discussed in the section on "Work of the Heart Under Static Load," the administration of β-blockers to a hypertensive weight lifter would be desirable for valid health reasons.

The other aspects of energy generation are clearly affected. This is true both for energy generation from the oxidative process and for lactic acid production. Before these negative effects are discussed below in detail, one may ask why such a discussion is necessary in the first place. Why should a *marathon runner* take β-blockers at all, if these drugs have potentially negative results? In this context we must repeat that in the young there may be legitimate indications for β-blocker therapy. The question is asked frequently whether a hypertensive marathon runner or *bicycle racer,* or a *swimmer* with arrhythmias, can continue their athletic activities under the therapeutic influence of β-blockers.

As indicated above, the β-blockers affect the reactions due to physical exercise not only on the cardiocirculatory system, but also in the area of metabolism. These last-mentioned relationships, which have been recognized only recently, must be discussed in relationship to the subject of the heart and sports because the introduction of the *cardioselective β-blockers* for the first time permit manipulation of the sympathetic system. The discussion of the clinical usefulness of cardioselectivity focused precisely on the importance of these drugs for the physically active patient treated with β-blockers.

The effect of the β-blockers on the adaptation of *cardiac function* under exercise can be best demonstrated by studying the *pulse rate.* The depression in the rate is much more marked under exercise than at rest. This becomes increasingly obvious as the intensity of the load increases. The difference between the observed heart rate and the presumptive heart rate continues to widen as the intensity of the load increases (Fig 6–2). The inadequate heart rate adaptation forces the heart to use compensatory mechanisms. In the healthy heart this is accomplished by an increased *stroke volume*, even though the contractility of the heart is diminished (see Fig 3–16). Our own corresponding data are presented in Figure 6–3. Similar observations were also made by other authors such as Lund-Johansen. An increase in stroke volume in spite of reduced contractility assumes the presence of a functioning *Starling mechanism*. On the other hand, it must be recognized that under β-blockade the work of the heart is decreased in spite of identical total physical work, since the blood pressure increase does not need to be quite as high (Fig 6–4).

In the presence of preexisting myocardial injury such an increase in stroke volume may no longer be possible. Studies in hospital patients show that in the β-blocked patient the stroke volume remains constant or even decreases during exercise (Blümchen, 1981; Lichtlen, 1969). The activation of the Starling mechanism leads to a decrease in coronary artery perfusion because of the rise in end-diastolic ventricular pressure. In spite of this negative effect, the reaction in rate and contractility as well as in pressure tips the scales in favor of the therapy by reducing the oxygen requirements even for the coronary patient. This can be shown very well on the stress ECG (Fig 6–5).

In the athletically active man, β-blockade reduces the maximal possible rate and contractility and thus limits the *rate* and *contractility reserves*. This was pointed out particularly by Roskamm (1972). The exercise tolerance of the normal heart is thus clearly restricted under maximal demands. In the high-performance athlete, there is a danger of car-

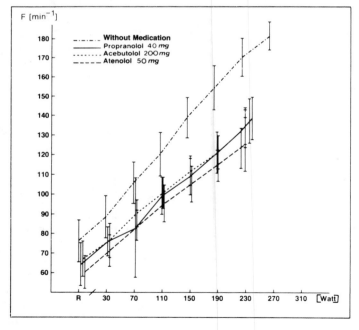

FIG 6–2.

The effect of beta-receptor blockers on the heart rate under load conditions. Twelve students were studied, first under control conditions and then under the effect of 40 mg propranolol, 200 mg acebutolol, and 50 mg atenolol. The loss in rate increase becomes more evident as the load increases. The rate deficit spreads like the blades of a pair of scissors.

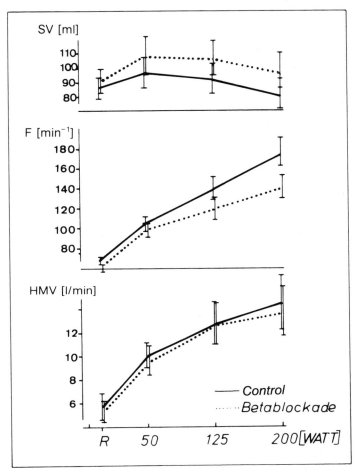

FIG 6–3.
Effect of 40 mg propranolol on hemodynamics under load conditions. The studies were performed on five healthy males by the dye-dilution technique. While the cardiac output does not change significantly, the stroke volume must be greater in view of the lower heart rate.

diac dilatation under maximal load. We have occasionally observed the appearance of cardiac complaints (dyscardias, premature beats) under β-blockade and after maximal loads. Another potential danger to the athlete lies in the possibility of a nonphysiologic cardiac enlargement under persistent forced activity and in the presence of a stroke volume considerably larger than normal.

The negative effects of the β-blockers on energy generation affect both the fat and glycogen values. Each of these is governed by a different receptor. While lipolysis is largely controlled by β_1-receptors, glycolysis and glycogenolysis are differentially controlled in the muscle by β_2-receptors and in the liver by α-receptors (Carlström, 1970; William-Olsson, 1979). *Long range endurance is determined by* the glycogen reserves in muscle that can be only partially replaced by fat. Under β-blockade, therefore, the energy generation from glycogen becomes even more important.

On the basis of this receptor model, it

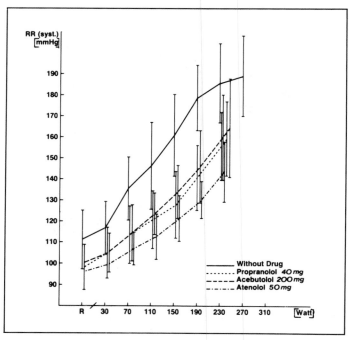

FIG 6–4.

Effect of various beta-receptor blockers on the systolic pressure under load conditions. The studies were performed according to the plan described in Figure 6–2.

seems appropriate to use primarily cardioselective drugs in patients who have to undergo physical exercise or in athletes who have to be started on β-blockers. As stated above, the cardioselective group interferes less with the utilization of muscle glycogen. This was pointed out very forcibly in Germany by Franz and Lohmann (1979), who have found an alarming drop in blood sugar during physical stress in patients on the nonselective β-blocker pindolol. There was no drop when the selective β-blockers acebutolol or metoprolol were used. This is in agreement with reports in the literature that describe severe *hypoglycemia* in patients running the marathon under β-blocker therapy (Holm, 1981).

It is true, however, that these reports are not unanimous. In more recent studies using the same design, Dorow (1982) was unable to duplicate the above results. The studies of Lundborg (1981)

have shown that there was indeed an interruption in energy liberation from glycogen and a drop in serum glucose level in persons on β-blockers under long-term load conditions. This response was more pronounced with nonselective β-blockers than with selective ones. It is also true, however, that decreases in blood sugar levels, significantly different from those seen in placebo controls, occurred only when the exercise period was extensive (at least 1 hour).

Our own studies comparing a series of cardioselective and nonselective β-blockers (acebutolol, atenolol, metoprolol, pindolol, and propranolol) were unable to demonstrate a significant superiority for the cardioselective blockers. After an exercise period lasting one hour, we found no advantage in using cardioselective blockers in a group of healthy physical education students (Fig 6–6). Similar studies in *diabetics* (Fig 6–7)

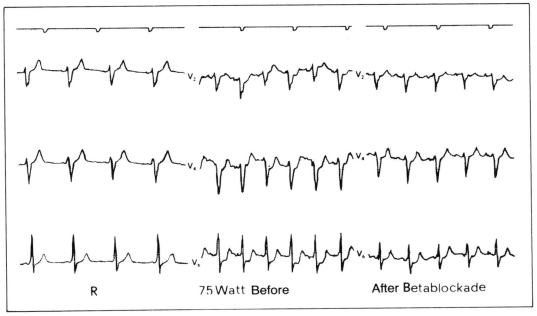

R　　　　　　　75 Watt **Before**　　　　　　　**After Betablockade**

FIG 6–5.
Effect of a beta-receptor blockade on a pathologic stress electrocardiogram. The ECG is unremarkable at rest in a coronary artery patient *(left)*. At 75 watt load, repolarization abnormalities appear that would have denied admission of this patient to a coronary artery activity club. After administration of a beta-receptor blocker the stress ECG returns to normal *(right)* and the exercise tolerance is clearly improved.

showed a greater drop in blood sugar during exercise in patients on propranolol, when compared to patients on the cardioselective β-blockers, acebutolol and atenolol.

The metabolic effects of the β-blockers can also be demonstrated by measuring *lactic acid production*. As shown in Figure 6–8, during moderate exercise the β-blockers lead to a slight decrease in the lactic acid levels. The maximal lactic acid concentration is also less when compared to a control group. There are two possible explanations for this observation. One explanation would relate the lower levels of lactic acid to a decreased production of this substance, since glycolysis is also stimulated by the catecholamines. The other explanation is based on the findings of Holmberg (1979) who suggested, on the basis of muscle biopsies, that the decreased blood levels of lactic acid were due to a decreased wash-out of lactic acid from the muscles. This in turn may be the result of a decreased *peripheral perfusion* caused by the β-blockers. This is in agreement with the frequent complaints of athletes on β-blockers about a variety of *muscle problems* during exercise. Regardless of the explanation of this hitherto unexplained phenomenon, a disturbance in energy generation from lactic acid must lead to a decrease in the performance of some athletes such as *the 400 m runners*.

In summarizing the discussion on the effects of the β-blockers on the *performance of athletes* the following can be said:

1. In those forms of athletics which are largely determined by psychologic factors, the β-blockers may be helpful.

2. In other forms of athletics such as power sports and rapid-power sports,

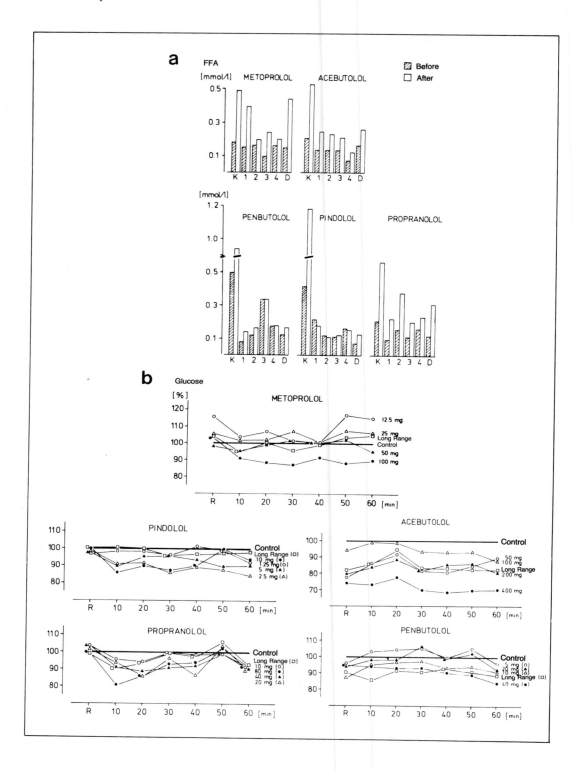

there is no evidence to date that β-blockers decrease performance.

3. In those forms of athletics that require a maximal energy release from lactic acid or from oxydation, the β-blockers decrease performance.

The athlete is also at some risk in the cardiac area and from the eventual appearance of hypoglycemia. For this reasons, extreme long-term exercises must be discouraged under β-blockade. As already discussed, it may be necessary to treat hypertensive performance athletes with drugs, specifically β-blockers. In view of the enormous demands made on the cardiocirculatory system and on metabolism by modern performance athletics, absolutely perfect health must be a precondition for participation. This precondition can obviously not be met by an athlete who has to take β-blockers.

4. In the athletes who insist on participating in intensive and long-term physical activity, in spite of the concerns expressed in No. 3 above, the use of cardioselective β-blockers may offer some advantage. These considerations cannot be applied to the physically active, average patient. For this person the advantages are purely theoretical, since the differences in the metabolic effects between the two groups of drugs are so small as to be meaningless.

5. There are some special groups of patients engaged in physical activity in whom the selective β-blockers may have an advantage. These are the diabetics who require β-blockers. In this group, however, the suppression of the warning signals of hypoglycemia by the β-blockers and the delay in recovery from hypoglycemia are serious concerns.

In the last section we had discussed the effects of the β-blockers on the *exercise tolerance* of the patient. This will be discussed further with special reference to the cardiocirculatory patients. In considering the relationship of β-blockers and physical exercise, there was a fear, particularly early in the development of β-blockers, that these may have a *negative effect* on each other. The partially negative inotropic effect of the β-blocking substances, the blockade of the adaptation mechanism of the heart to exercise-triggered sympathetic stimulation, and the earlier described utilization of the Starling mechanism inevitably led to a fear of triggering a cardiac *stress insufficiency* in a heart that because of its underlying disease was already functioning at the outer limits of its functional efficiency. Experience has shown in the

---

FIG 6–6.

The effect of various beta-receptor blockers on the substrates of energy metabolism under load conditions (performed in cooperation with Koebe, 1985). Five different β-blockers were studied: some cardioselective (metoprolol, acebutolol), and some nonselective (penbutolol, pindolol, propranolol). The studies were performed during a 1-hour load test at 50% of the maximal performance capacity. In each case six healthy physical education students were studied and the mean value of their performance was used for each β-blocker. The subjects had to perform the load test first without drug and then after 10, 20, 40, and 80 mg of propranolol. This was followed by a 4-week period on 40 mg propranolol. At the end of this time the load test was repeated. **a,** the effects on free fatty acids, before and after the load. The numbers *1* to *4* represent the four different dosage rates of the β-blocker. *D* is the result after the long-term study. It appears that the increase in free fatty acid that occurs in the control situation is almost completely suppressed by all the β-blockers used. **b,** the effects on serum glucose. The blood glucose level decreases slightly during load conditions after each of the β-blockers tested. The increased trend toward hypoglycemia reported in the literature in connection with the nonselective blockers was not seen in the present study.

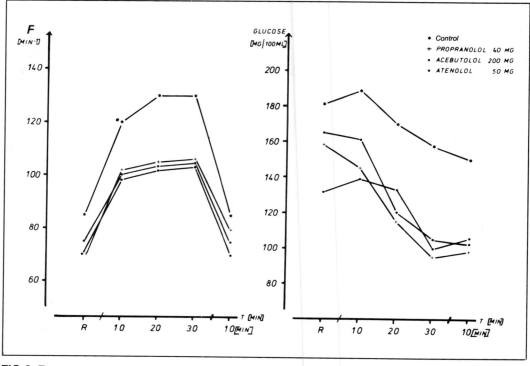

FIG 6–7.

The effect of physical load after beta-blockade in seven insulin-dependent diabetics (in cooperation with deRose, 1983). The load was applied for 30 minutes at 50% of maximal capacity. It is apparent that the nonselective blocker propranolol causes the least decrease in heart rate but the greatest drop in blood glucose. Two of the 7 subjects developed mild hypoglycemia under propranolol that was not seen under the two selective blockers, acebutolol and atenolol.

meantime that these fears were exaggerated. Even the postinfarct patient can engage in physical activity under β-blockade provided that he has sufficient myocardial reserve.

As stated above, the performance of the high-performance athlete is decreased by β-blockers, depending to some extent on the particular form of athletics involved. In the cardiocirculatory patient, the β-blockers tend to improve performance. One of the reasons for this is the fact that the cardiocirculatory patient, contrary to the high-performance athlete, should never be pushed to the limits of his endurance. The optimal training intensity for these patients is in the middle ranges of load conditions, where the limitations in pulse rate increases are of less significance. In addition, the cardiocirculatory patient cannot function to the full limits of his efficiency, since his exercise tolerance is already limited by the underlying disease process.

This problem area can be best illustrated by looking at the admission criteria for patients applying to the coronary artery activity clubs and that have been described in detail in the section on "Evaluation of Exercise Tolerance." The exercise tolerance of these patients is decreased when even moderate stress causes coronary artery insufficiency manifested as a *repolarization disturbance* (see Fig 6–5). If, in these cases, the oxygen balance is improved, the exercise tolerance should improve as well.

The same is true for the appearance

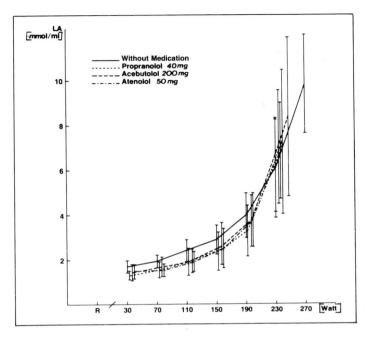

FIG 6–8.
The effect of beta-receptor blockers on serum lactate levels. The study was performed according to the model in Figure 6–2. In the submaximal region there is a slight decrease in lactate levels after all β-blockers. The lactic acid level rises somewhat more rapidly than under control conditions and the lines cross at one point. The aerobic-anaerobic threshold does not change. The maximal lactate level observed was lower under the influence of the β-blockers.

of alarming, *stress-induced arrhythmias.* To treat such arrhythmias, which certainly have increased sympathetic activity as an important etiologic component, the administration of β-blockers is a matter of course. In the individual case, however, a stress electrocardiogram (ECG) should always be performed under β-blockade, since the effectiveness of the antiarrhythmic medication can never be predicted with any certainty in any one individual. Our own studies suggest (Rost, 1981) that about two thirds of all exercise-induced premature beats respond well to β-blocker therapy. The response is better in supraventricular arrhythmias than in ventricular ones. It must be stated, however, that in some cases the arrhythmia is made worse by the drug-induced preponderance of the reentry mechanism. In all considerations of the relationship of drug therapy and

physical stress, the potential negative effects must be kept in mind.

A further limitation of exercise tolerance may be due to *excessive hypertension.* This type of exercise-induced hypertension also responds well to β-blocker therapy. Concerning the selection of the individual antihypertensive agent in the athlete-patient, the reader is referred to the section on "Functional Cardiocirculatory Diseases." In that section, the measures to improve exercise tolerance in functional circulatory disturbances are also discussed under the heading of the *hyperkinetic heart syndrome.*

Besides the question concerning the effects of β-blockers on performance, another question that is very important in practice concerns the problem of *changes in the response to stress* under the influence of the β-blockers. The most com-

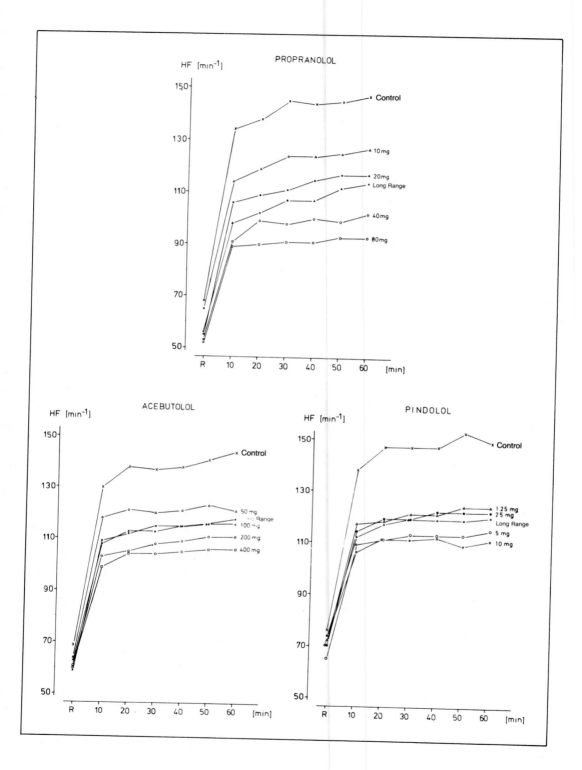

monly asked question in practice concerning the relationship of β-blockers and physical training is about the possibility to *correct the pulse rate* in the β-blocked patients.

In this matter, it is very difficult to come up with any general guidelines. The earlier discussion and the findings shown in Figure 6–2 indicate that the degree of rate decrease depends on the intensity of the exercise. It is further determined by the dose of the β-blocker and by individual factors. Figure 6–9 shows that with propranolol, the rate decrease is strongly dose-dependent. With the intrinsically acting β-blockers, the rate decrease is much less dose-dependent. These findings were duplicated by Kober (1982). Furthermore, the effect on the heart rate is highly dependent on individual factors.

The advice frequently given to β-blocked patients, namely to set their stress pulse rate at 20 to 25 beats below their normal training heart rate, is very simplistic. It is valid only for a moderate stress, corresponding to a pulse rate of 130, and for a moderate dose of β-blockers of perhaps 40 mg of propranolol. With more effective β-blockade the pulse correction must be raised. A dose of β-blocking drug, corresponding to 80 mg propranolol, decreases the pulse rate by about 30 beats per minute at moderate levels of stress.

Theoretically, every level of stress and every dose of β-blocker should have its own pulse correction factor. Experiential data, as those given above, will be reasonably satisfactory, if the investigator has access to only a limited number of β-blockers. Advice, which can be given in

this context, is to watch the *respirations.* As shown in Figure 6–8, the *lactic acid concentration curve* is considerably less affected by β-blockers than the pulse rate. This lactic acid curve shows a typical course. In mild stress the lactic acid level hardly rises at all. In the nontrained person at about two thirds of the individual maximal capacity, the serum lactic acid level rises sharply. This so-called *aerobic-anaerobic threshold* sets the limit where oxygen supply and utilization in the muscle are no longer optimal.

This threshold area can be viewed as the optimal goal of training. Greater loads lead to overexertion, lesser loads to underachievement. As shown in Figure 6–8, this threshold is not significantly affected by the β-blockers. Clinical observation of the patient under physical load makes an approximate determination of the threshold performance possible, since the sudden increase in lactic acid levels causes a marked respiratory stimulation. This gives the old, but mostly ignored, concept of using respiration as a guide to physical exercise a new hold on life. Observing the patient on a bicycle ergometer can determine the moment when hyperventilation begins. The level of performance, at this point, and the pulse rate, permit the physician to give the patient rather precise advice concerning optimal exercise. Even advice as simple as: "running without panting" or "run only so fast that you can still chat with your running mate" are practical, and scientifically sound.

As already indicated in the general introduction, the pulse rate is by no means the only autonomic function to change under physical exercise. Accord-

---

FIG 6–9.
The effect of different doses of three beta-blockers on the heart rate under load conditions. The studies were performed in cooperation with Koebe, as described in Figure 6–6. With propranolol there is a clear, dose-related decrease in heart rate. There is a dose-related decrease in heart rate after pindolol and acebutolol as well, but the decrease is very much less.

ing to our own studies (Rost, 1982), the volume of respiration is decreased under the influence of β-blockers. Sweating, on the other hand, may be significantly increased in some individuals by β-blockers under identical load conditions. The decrease of the reaction to hypoglycemia in the diabetic has already been mentioned.

Another question that is frequently asked in practice in connection with the β-blockers is: "What is the degree to which *training can be pushed,* when the pulse rate increases are limited by the beta blockers?" In a recent study, Sable (1982) found that in the patient under total autonomic blockade, consisting of atropine and very large doses of β-blockers, training had no effects at all. It seems clear, therefore, that a functional sympathetic drive is necessary to achieve the goals of any training effort. On the other hand, this study does not rule out the possibility that no training effects are possible under β-blockade, since the doses used in the study were far larger than the customary therapeutic range (up to 640 mg of propranolol per day). One of our co-workers (Liesen, 1971) found that under clinically customary doses of propranolol, an improvement of performance could be achieved with training.

OTHER CARDIOCIRCULATORY DRUGS

For the reasons mentioned, there are a number of reviews dealing with the relationship between the β-blockers and athletics. Data dealing with the relationship of athletics and the other drugs are scattered far and wide in the pharmacologic, physiologic, and clinical literature. For many drugs taken by physically active patients, there is no reference at all. If any reference can be found, it deals almost exclusively with acute observations. Yet the effects of these drugs could be

quite different on chronic administration, as is well known for the β-blockers. The studies of Lohmann (1981) have shown that the β-blockers will interfere with lipolysis under stress on an acute basis. Under chronic use, this decrease in lipolysis is compensated for by a noncatecholamine dependent metabolic pathway. In view of this unsatisfactory state of affairs, it is very difficult to gain any overview on the effects of the other cardiocirculatory drugs on physical exercise. In the following paragraphs an attempt will be made to indicate some of the effects that the drugs most commonly prescribed for the cardiocirculatory patients have on exercise tolerance.

Of all the cardiocirculatory drugs that are taken by physically active patients, *digitalis* was, and remains, the most important, at least in Germany. As Figure 6–1 shows, 60% of our own patients, in our own coronary artery activity club, took some form of digitalis preparation in 1979. This is in spite of the fact that this is a highly selected and carefully monitored group. Recently this percentage decreased significantly. Nevertheless, it could be assumed that in many of these patients digitalization is unnecessary. It is therefore essential to reemphasize at this time that digitalis improves the pumping functions of the heart, particularly of the failing myocardium. This is true under exercise as well. The hemodynamic studies of Williams (1958) showed that cardiac output decreased, rather than increased, in healthy, digitalized experimental subjects under identical load conditions. Since the blood pressure did not change, Williams assumed that the change was due to an increase in peripheral resistance, i.e., a vascular response. In contrast to this, the exercise tolerance of the patients who have a cardiac insufficiency at rest and under stress is improved by digitalis.

Even in the coronary artery patient, there is no indication for digitalization, unless there is also evidence of *myocardial insufficiency*. Stress angina is improved only if there is a simultaneous stress insufficiency. In this situation, digitalization decreases the filling pressure and the size of the heart. The decreased mural tension results in decreased oxygen requirement and thus in better oxygen balance. In contrast, the increased *contractility* of the heart and the increased peripheral resistance produced by digitalis may lead to a decrease in exercise tolerance in the coronary patient who does not also have a myocardial insufficiency.

A decrease in exercise tolerance under digitalis can occasionally be attributed to an increased tendency toward *stress-induced arrhythmias*. Gooch (1974) found that in 20 patients who had clear signs of digitalization on the resting ECG, arrhythmias appeared on the stress ECG. Digitalis, therefore, can improve exercise tolerance in the patient with myocardial insufficiency, but can decrease exercise tolerance in patients with other types of heart disease.

Of particular interest are the changes in the *stress-induced reactions*. Here the effects on *pulse rate* are less significant. In patients with myocardial insufficiency, the increase in *pulse rate* after digitalization will be less apparent in view of the general improvement of cardiac performance. If, however, healthy volunteers or coronary patients, whose myocardial function is well compensated, are digitalized, particularly with the currently commonly used digoxin preparations, the pulse rate will be lowered less than 10 beats per minute under similar load conditions. In this connection the effect of digitalis on the *stress ECG* is worthy of mention. It is well known that under digitalis the stress ECG may show ST segment depressions that cannot be attributed to coronary artery insufficiency, and that may give rise to false positive interpretations. On the other hand, it has been pointed out (Lehmann, 1979) that such changes occur to a significant degree only in patients with significant coronary artery disease who are digitalized. Nevertheless, ignoring the changes due to digitalis may lead to an incorrect assessment of the exercise tolerance of these patients. A good example for this is shown in Figure 6–10. Here, after digitalization, repolarization disturbances appear already after 75-watt loads, and disappear on withdrawal studies. The exercise tolerance in these patients is clearly better than what would have been assumed if the effects of medication had been ignored. The evaluation of the stress ECG under the influence of digitalization will not be discussed further, and the reader is referred to an earlier monograph (Rost, 1982).

An interesting and important perspective is gained from an examination of the relationship between physical activity and the *anticoagulants*. Numerous coronary artery patients are on anticoagulants. In the groups monitored by us, a review revealed an incidence of 60% in 1979. Since that time, a developing scepticism concerning the value of long term anticoagulation has decreased this number. Anticoagulants are of particular importance in the physically-active patient after valve replacement, as discussed in the section on "Exercise Tolerance in the Patient With Cardiac Lesions, After Surgical Correction." In selecting an appropriate form of athletics in the anticoagulated patient, particular attention must be paid to the possibility of hemorrhagic complications. The anticoagulated patient, particularly the patient who is dependent on effective anticoagulation, must avoid all forms of athletics where the risks of injury are high. These include downhill skiing, riding, and contact sports like soccer. Even in the framework of the coronary artery club activities, the athletic instructor must be aware of this problem and must avoid the situations

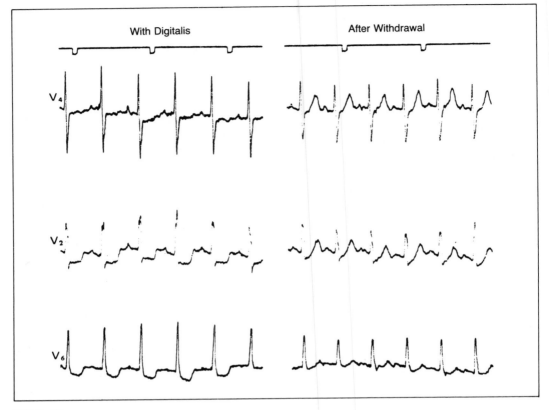

FIG 6–10.
The effect of digitalis on the stress electrocardiogram (ECG). In a coronary artery patient significant repolarization disturbances appeared on the stress ECG *(left)*. On a withdrawal trial they no longer appear *(right)*. If the pharmacologic effects had been ignored, this patient's exercise tolerance would have been set at an improper level.

where this risk is appreciable. For details, the reader is referred to the section on "Evaluation of the Various Athletic Activities From the Perspective of the Coronary Artery Patient." By giving serious consideration to these principles, we have seen no serious hemorrhagic complications in the Cologne coronary artery activity club during the 10 years that it has been under our supervision. To date, there is no information concerning any possible difference between patients on Coumadin and patients on antiplatelet-aggregation drugs.

An interesting aspect of the *synergistic effects* of physical training and drug therapy can be demonstrated in relationship to the anticoagulants. Physical train-

ing also affects the coagulation mechanism. The few, and yet inconclusive, data suggest that physical activity enhances thrombopoiesis and the aggregation of thrombocytes while it also activates the fibrinolytic system (Böhmer, 1974; Haber, 1980; Metze, 1981; Rieger, 1981).

It seems that the increased coagulability appears only under extreme load conditions. Sudden deaths in young athletes were attributed to coronary artery thrombosis due to increased coagulability. Samek (1982) reported an increased incidence of coagulopathies in young patients who developed an acute infarct under physical stress in the absence of any coronary artery disease.

On the other hand, it has been argued

that the increased fibrinolytic activity seen under physical load conditions may be important in the prevention of secondary complications of arteriosclerotic coronary artery disease. This reveals a synergistic effect between training and anticoagulation.

Among the *coronary artery drugs* other than the β-blockers, the *nitrate preparations* deserve particular mention. As is well known, the nitrate preparations are particularly active on the peripheral vascular system. The decrease in peripheral resistance leads to a decrease in the so-called afterload, i.e., the arterial pressure. Venous dilatation, i.e., venous pooling, or internal phlebotomy, reduces the cardiac output and the preload. In this way both the volume work and the pressure work of the heart are decreased.

Similar hemodynamic responses, well known under resting conditions, can be demonstrated under load conditions as well. Nordenfelt and Westling (1967) could show these responses even better when sublingual nitroglycerin was used. With a 50-watt load, the *cardiac output* decreased by an order of magnitude of 1.4 L/minute. With higher loads, the decrease was even more marked. The reduction in cardiac output was accompanied by a marked increase in *heart rate,* so that *the stroke volume* was also decreased. The systolic pressure decreased by 14 mm Hg, while the diastolic pressure remained unchanged. The same observations were made in normal volunteers as well as in cardiac patients.

The effect of the *long-acting nitrates* is along the same lines, but considerably less marked. The studies of Jansen (1982) and Beautefau (1980) showed that the heart rate was not affected under exercise. The latter author found no changes in pressure either, while Jansen, in a study with a mononitrate, found the same pressure relationships as Nordenfelt (1967). On the other hand, Jansen found no appreciable effect on the cardiac output and stroke volume.

Numerous studies, summarized by Jansen, show an *improvement in exercise tolerance* in coronary artery patients on ergometer tests. This is true both for the intensity and the duration of the exercise. The determining factor appears to be the decrease in *pulmonary artery pressure* and the ensuing decrease in diastolic filling, which, in turn, allows better coronary perfusion. There appears to be no direct effect on coronary perfusion, even under exercise. Another point that improves exercise tolerance is a decrease in peripheral resistance and thus of the pressure work of the heart. According to Powles (1981), the prolongation of the ejection time under the influence of nitrates is also of positive value for exercise tolerance. The same author also reports a decrease in the tendency for arrhythmias.

A significant disadvantage of the nitrates lies in the development of *tolerance.* The data of Jansen show clearly that in the long-term studies there is distinctly less decrease in pulmonary artery pressure than in acute experiments. Another disadvantage of the nitrates is the *nitrate headache,* which, according to our observations, is an important side effect under exercise. Physical education students participating in an acute experiment on the effects of *isosorbide dinitrate* and physical exercise developed such severe nitrate headaches that the experiment had to be cancelled. The increase in pulse rate and the decrease in blood pressure were significant in these studies.

The third important group that must be mentioned in connection with the coronary artery patients are the *calcium antagonists.* This group contains widely differing substances. It includes, as extreme examples, *nifedipine,* which acts primarily on the vascular system, and *verapamil,* effective particularly as an antiarrhythmic agent. The third representative of the calcium antagonists is *diltiazem,* which is of clinical importance and that is pharmacologically between nifedipine and verapamil.

Their effectiveness in the treatment of angina pectoris is due primarily to the arterial vasodilator effect, which is a common property of all the agents in this group. This effect leads to a decrease in peripheral resistance and at the same time to a dilatation of the large, epicardial coronary arteries. Much of the discussion currently centers on their effect on the functional narrowing of the coronary arteries, the so-called *dynamic coronary artery stenosis*. This is a condition where a spastic component is superimposed on an underlying arteriosclerotic change.

Contrary to the nitrates, which lead to a decrease in cardiac output under load conditions, the calcium antagonists, which act on the vessels, cause an increase in *cardiac output*. Our own studies have demonstrated this, as far as nifedipine is concerned (Hollmann, 1975). This difference in the effect of the nitrates and the calcium antagonists rests on the fact that the calcium antagonists are effective primarily on the arterial side. Venous pooling, if it occurs at all, is only of very minor significance. The increase in cardiac output is accomplished by a combination of an increase in heart rate (5–10 beats per minute), and a slight increase in stroke volume. The *increase in heart rate* is so small that not all authors have been able to demonstrate it.

While an increase in heart rate under stress is considered unfavorable from the point of view of myocardial oxygen demand, and since these two parameters are tightly linked to each other, practical experience has shown that the exercise tolerance of the coronary artery patients is distinctly improved by the calcium antagonists. This can be proven by stress ECG studies. Obviously the factors that improve the oxygen balance, i.e., improved coronary artery perfusion and a decrease in peripheral resistance, outweigh the effects of the heart rate. The calcium antagonists that act on the cardiac rhythm, such as verapamil (Pozenel, 1981), diltiazem (Hossack, 1981; Kober, 1981), and the less widely used fendilin (our own observations), all lower the submaximal heart rate to only a negligible degree.

The *blood pressure* is slightly decreased under the calcium antagonists, when equal load conditions are compared in normotensive patients. This decrease of about 10 mm Hg for each load level was demonstrated by us for nifedipine, and by Pozenel (1981) for verapamil. More recently, the calcium antagonists are being seriously considered as effective therapy for *hypertension*. One of the factors that may lead to improved exercise tolerance under the antiarrhythmic calcium antagonists is their ability to suppress the appearance of *stress-induced cardiac arrhythmias*.

As far as the question of the effects of the calcium antagonists on *performance* is concerned, it seems that in healthy persons there is no such effect. We found no change in the *maximal oxygen uptake* in physical education students under nifedipine and fendilin. In contrast to the β-blockers, this lack of effect is probably due to a lack in producing a significant rate decrease under load conditions. In coronary artery patients the exercise tolerance is improved by all the calcium antagonists by improving the myocardial oxygen balance. Such an improvement in exercise tolerance can be expected when the negative effects of stress-induced arrhythmias or excessive hypertension are controlled by these drugs. From the point of view of exercise tolerance, the calcium antagonists have definite advantages over the beta blockers.

The increasing importance of the calcium antagonists in the treatment of hypertension gives us an opportunity to lead into a discussion of the *antihypertensive drugs* in general. In this context we can refer to the calcium antagonists discussed above and the β-blockers discussed earlier. These latter drugs are assuming a major role in the management of hypertension. The problems of the pharmacologically treated hypertensive patient engaging in athletic activity has been discussed in the section on "Hypertension."

The next important group in the management of hypertension that must be mentioned are the *diuretics*. As already mentioned, Franz (1979) found that they had no effect on stress hypertension. According to the review of Powles (1981), there is evidence that hydrochlorothiazide and chlorthalidon decrease the stress hypertension; the former, by decreasing peripheral resistance, and the latter, by decreasing cardiac output. In view of the very numerous and very different diuretic substances used in therapy, all we can say at this time is that the effect of these substances on the stress responses of hypertensive patients must be investigated. Particular attention must be paid in these studies to the problem of dose-dependent responses. Our own studies with furosemide, mefruside, triamterene, and bemetizide have shown that in healthy volunteers, after oral administration the maximal oxygen uptake is not decreased. The last two drugs led to a significant decrease in the serum potassium levels and to a significant increase in uric acid. The loss of electrolytes and the increase in uric acid that may lead to the formation of kidney stones in the long-distance runner are definite disadvantages.

There are very few data concerning the many other types of drugs that are used in the treatment of hypertension. These are collected in the review by Powles (1981). Hydralazine as a vasodilator affects the smooth muscles directly. It causes a reflex tachycardia and an increase in cardiac output, which may be undesirable under load conditions (Moyer, 1953). Alpha-methyldopa, a competitive blocker of noradrenaline as a transmitter substance, causes a marked decrease in heart rate under load conditions (Sannerstedt, 1970). The data concerning the effects on exercise cardiac output are inconclusive, since both increases and decreases have been reported.

Clonidine decreases the peripheral sympathetic tone by stimulating the central α-receptors. This leads to a definite decrease in circulating catecholamines (Hansen, 1981). This also leads to a decrease in heart rate. Since the cardiac output does not change appreciably, the stroke volume must increase (Onesti, 1971). Hansen claims that under stress increased noradrenaline increasingly replaces clonidine from the central receptors. This explains why this substance is much less effective under exercise than at rest.

Guanethidine, which acts as an adrenergic neuronal blocker, decreases the amount of stored catecholamines. This causes a marked decrease in heart rate, cardiac output, and stroke volume under stress. Under exercise this may lead to undesirable, severe hypotensive conditions (Dollery, 1961; Kahler, 1962).

To date there are no data on the newer antihypertensives, *prazosine* and *minoxidil*, as far as their effects on physical exercise are concerned.

As far as the *antiarrhythmic* drugs are concerned, the reader is referred to the earlier discussions on β-blockers and calcium antagonists. There are so few data concerning the effects of the numerous new and old drugs in this group on premature beats or stress hemodynamics that even a superficial review would be premature at this time.

Index